the

skin

nerd

Jennifer Rock is an award-winning skin lecturer and a multi-award winning dermal facialist and aesthetician. She is the founder of The Skin Nerd online skin consultancy and creator of the Cleanse Off Mitt® makeup removal tool.

Jennifer realised her passion for skin health when she was brought for her first facial by her mother at the tender age of thirteen. After years of working as a skin therapist – lecturing worldwide alongside renowned dermatologists such as Dr. Marc Ronert of IMAGE Skincare and Dr. Ahmar Khan, co-creator of the London Harley Street Medical Hospital – and being the brand ambassador for multiple cosmeceutical skincare brands, she became The Skin Nerd, using social media to get skinformation out there, sometimes through the medium of song. Her mantra is 'The skin is an organ – respect it accordingly'.

Nowadays, you'll find her standing at the helm of The Skin Nerd HQ, on television, in the pages of well-known publications and speaking on the radio.

Her end goal is to put as many people as possible on the road to skin health.

Website: www.theskinnerd.com
Instagram: @theskinnerdire
Twitter: @theskinnerdire
Facebook: The Skin Nerd Jennifer Rock

the
skin
nerd

Jennifer Rock

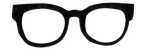

HACHETTE
BOOKS
IRELAND

First published in Ireland in 2018 by
HACHETTE BOOKS IRELAND

2

Cataloguing in Publication Data is available from the British Library

ISBN 9781473680517

Book design and typesetting by Anú Design, Tara

Printed in Italy by L.E.G.O. S.p.A

Hachette Books Ireland policy is to use papers that are natural, renewable and recyclable
products and made from wood grown in sustainable forests. The logging and manufacturing
processes are expected to conform to the environmental regulations of the country of origin.

Hachette Books Ireland
8 Castlecourt Centre
Castleknock
Dublin 15, Ireland

A division of Hachette UK Ltd
Carmelite House, 50 Victoria Embankment, EC4Y 0DZ

www.hachettebooksireland.ie

*The information found in this book is for general information purposes only and
should not be used as a substitute for medical or other professional advice. If you
are suffering from a skin or other medical condition that may require diagnosis and
treatment, we recommend that you seek the advice of a doctor.*

Contents

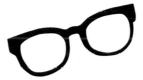

I nerdily wish to dedicate this book
to the gentleman and beautiful hooman who encouraged me
to be book-smart from an early age.

Diligent, meticulous, articulate,
a consummate professional — all while showing limitless
love and patience. My true mentor, you inspire me daily.
I love you always x

Introduction

Greetings, nerds.

New to my ways? Take no offence, the term is meant kindly.

What defines a 'skin nerd', I hear you ask?

A skin nerd is not just someone who wants healthy skin and makes it their mission. It's someone who places an emphasis on education, ingredients and science above marketing – someone who actively tries to understand what they're putting onto their skin and how it will work for their concerns. A skin nerd is someone who chastises their friends annoyingly about their face wipe usage, who would prefer to leave the house knickerless than without sunscreen. Someone who respects the skin as an organ. If you don't do this already, you will by the end of this book. I promise.

So, welcome, one and all, new and existing nerds to my big fat juicy book – a skincare bible, if I do say so myself. Followers of The Skin Nerd will know that for me – Jennifer Rock, the biggest nerd of all – this book has been a long time coming. It only took me ten years to get here, but condensing over a decade's worth of information, advice and opinion into one reliable guide was always going to be a task and a half (that said, it's been totally worth it).

For those unfamiliar with me, I am a beauty therapist and lecturer by qualification; a true nerd by genetics. Skin is my passion, love, career and distraction all rolled into one. I have been lucky enough to learn from the best in the world, to win facialist and training awards on an international level, and to lecture alongside plastic surgeons, nutritionists and aesthetic surgeons.

For as long as I can remember, it's been my dream to spread the word of good skin health across the globe. From developing a relationship with clients on a personal level when I started out, to broadening that community enormously across Snapchat, Instagram and, of course, via TheSkinNerd.com, putting pen to paper was always going to be the inevitable next step for me.

Those who follow me on social media will know of my hectic lifestyle (no, literally, I need to force myself to go to bed sometimes – not so good for the skin). From morning to night, I'm sharing what I've learned and what I practise myself with clients, whether that's at a live event or from the comfort of my PJs and spectacles at home.

But as an avid social-media user, with a business, a family and a life of my own, I know it can all get a little overwhelming – the sheer volume of information coming at us from all angles and the multitude of apps and advertisements that demand our attention from one end of the day to the other can be exhausting. This is especially true when it comes to skincare and it can be hard to see the wood from the trees and know what's actually helpful and what's nothing more than a marketing tactic. Not to mention the pressure a lot of us feel to have flawless skin in real life, without the help of an Instagram filter.

What I've observed over the past decade is that people don't know how or what to use on their skin or who to trust in skincare. Typically, if you approach a salon, they will sell you the brand they stock. This is the extent of their options, and therefore yours as a client. Similarly, a department store employee is on commission to advise on that one brand alone – which may or may not be ideal for your skin.

How will you know if what you are getting is just a paid-for opinion?

Where do you go for skin results rather than a fluffy puffy spa treatment?

How will you know when a massive brand has spent more money on their marketing and celebrity endorsements than the all-important research and development required to produce top-quality skincare?

It's tricky, but I'm here to set you on the straight and narrow.

Some dub me the 'Simon Cowell of skincare'. White shirt? Check. High-waisted pants? Check. Hairy chest? Not so much. Ultimately, I get this comparison because I am so downright appalled at the number of lies and yarns being fed in this industry that I tend to be frank and straight to the point in my answers. Skincare recommendations should be made by people with true knowledge of the skin's physiology, as well as insight into the psychological effects of skin problems. You deserve nothing less.

A word of warning – the rants may continue, but I am here to help. I know what I'm talking about and, by the end of this book, you will also know exactly what to look for and what to avoid.

And so, with a considerable bee in my bonnet and after an incredibly rewarding (but equally bananas) year of getting The Skin Nerd online consultancy clinic and skin store up and running, I wanted to slow right down for a minute (a long one), distilling everything I know – and everything you need to know – into something physical that you can hold in your hands.

I wanted to create a guide with which you could curl up and get stuck in – green-tea and stress-free environment essential – or leave glued to your bedside table or throw in your handbag as you make your way in the world. I wanted to create something you could take your time with in our fast-paced lives, something packed to the brim with exclusive Skinformation – you'll have to get used to my lingo; even my teenage son, aka Mini Nerd, speaks in 'skinisms' and 'nerdisms' – and my ultimate guide to Skingredients.

I also wanted to clear up some myths – the *ifs* and *buts* of skincare – once and for all. My aim is not only to help you achieve glorious skin, but also to save your hard-earned money and help you avoid stress in the long run. With so much science and hyperbole out there, I wanted to create something that is easy to read and as accessible as your favourites on Netflix.

For me, when educating people about their skin, there's a fine balance between having an incredibly dense, physiologically guided rant and a wishy-washy spiel that leaves you none the wiser. I try to make learning about the skin as engaging and fun as possible, while, at the same time, being informative. That said, I am The Skin Nerd, and to fully understand our skin and what it needs, the science part is essential.

My aim with this book – and with The Skin Nerd business on the whole – is to educate and empower everyone on what their skin is and what their skin needs to be healthy. And to offer you a helping hand as you take your first steps on a new path towards skin health. Ultimately, this book is about shouting from the rooftops that the skin is an organ – I'll be repeating this ad nauseum, working in the Skindustry for so long has shown me that so many people do not realise this – and, as an organ, your skin must be respected accordingly.

Within the covers of this book, you'll find the Nerdie stance on what the skin needs, what makes it tick and precisely what you should be doing to target your specific skin concerns. You'll find out what to expect from your skin as the ageing process takes its course, how to handle the blemishes that get us all from time to time, and exactly how your skin works from the inside out. I want to empower those of you who feel down and helpless about your skin to realise that, with a bit of Nerdie knowledge and some personal effort, you *can* have healthy skin.

But don't expect any fluff. What you're getting here is my honest, expert and backed-by-science opinion (that, sometimes, you won't want to hear) and plenty of practical, BS-free info on ingredients, products and trends, as well as education on the skin itself. Terminology that might be tricky has been highlighted in blue and you can jump straight to the glossary for an explanation of these words.

Now we need to talk about what this book won't do.

There are plenty of books and online resources that claim to offer a quick-fix solution, leaving you with baby-butt skin for the rest of your life – this book isn't one of them.

This book will not fix your skin. You will fix your skin. Step 1 is taking action.

This is a truth that must be told. Instead, a combination of the advice within this book and a thorough skincare consultation is what will bring about the most impactful changes. You can start with theskinnerd.com online consultation and, if you need to be directed to a dermatologist or doctor, you will be. Everyone's skincare journey is personal, or as we call it 'skindividual', and a proactive and preventative attitude will bring your skin to optimal health.

This book will not give you recipes for body scrubs, honey-based face masks that you'd rather eat than apply to your skin, or references to products that I do not believe will help your skin in some way or another.

If you are an avid spot picker or a wipes user or someone who sleeps with their makeup on, steel yourself for some bad news, my nerd. What's more, although, at this moment, you may believe that what you put inside your body does not affect your skin, you absolutely won't believe this when you've reached the last page of this book. But this is a good thing!

Though I know you may want a quick fix – don't we all – I am not offering one sexy solution nor am I going to show you how to throw the kitchen sink at your skin only to make things worse. I am going to be real, honest and unbiased.

Personally, I've always taken an impartial approach to skincare. I firmly believe that when it comes to products, you won't find what I believe to be the core concepts and skingredients in one range alone; I don't believe it's been created yet. Every single person's skin is unique and thus comes with unique concerns that must be treated with a bespoke regime.

The Skin Nerd approach to skin focuses on guidance, which I believe should be plentiful, accessible and long term. Having a skin guide means that your routine can be changed when an aspect of your life changes – such as if you become pregnant or find yourself struggling with stress that affects your skin – and that you will never fall foul of the law of not over-exfoliating (more on that later).

I believe in a 360° approach to skin health.

This means treating your skin from the inside with nutrition and supplements, and on the outside with topical skincare, SPF and mineral makeup. This book will inform you thoroughly on each part of this approach.

I do not believe in a one-and-done method because everything has an impact on the skin – the environment, your wellbeing, your diet, your age, your hormones, your bad habits and your good habits. As you read this book, I hope you'll be inspired to make lifestyle changes, not just skincare changes. What's more, I hope you will learn that your skin is not merely an accessory or something to make you look good, it's a barometer of your internal health.

How Should You Read This Book?

Depending on your level of knowledge already, this can be a dip-in and dip-out kinda book. But, wherever you find yourself, I strongly advise that you start with the first few chapters, and wrap your head around, or at least refresh, your anatomy and physiology knowledge, so that you really understand the skin and how it works. This will also help you get on board with The Skin Nerd approach, principles and philosophies.

Then, you might prefer to jump straight to a concern that you have right now, such as how stress affects skin (because, boy, that is a biggie). If acne is just not on your radar, you might skip past that and come back to it later on. Just don't assume that a lack of spots means your skin is healthy, or that what you put into your body or onto your skin won't lead to breakouts down the line. That is like believing all slender 'hoomans' (humans) are healthy.

This is not a book that you should read once and file away to gather dust, it's something that you should come back to again and again to help you hone your skincare routine as life takes you in different directions.

Are you ready to embrace the 360° Nerdie philosophy and do the work necessary to get the skin you've always wanted?

Great.

But first … homework. STOP – contain your excitement.

Your Skin Diary

At this point, I want to introduce the idea of a skin diary. Start this now, today, and I promise that navigating your way towards skin health will become a whole lot easier. This book can show you the way, but only you – with a pen and paper and unwavering honesty – can track your skin, in the same way you might record a food diary to suss out your food intolerances.

It's important to get very familiar with how your skin behaves, how it reacts and how your lifestyle is having an impact on it. This is crucial. All will be explored in greater detail throughout the book but, for now, I've listed below what should be considered in your personal skin diary.

Also, I always suggest taking a photo on day one, then two weeks later, two weeks after that, and so on to track how your skin changes. If we are taking photos daily, we run into obsessive territory and that's not helpful either. You will also notice differences in a two-week period more easily, whereas day to day, it's harder and you may just drive yourself bananas.

You should record all of the following notes at night-time in one go. Observe how your skin looks and feels each day.

Lifestyle

1. ## How much sleep you're getting. Why?

    Sleep affects the skin regeneration process and healing ability. Seven hours is the ideal amount of sleep for optimally performing skin, but the key is quality sleep. If you wake up feeling rested, rather than irritable and groggy, you are getting good sleep that's beneficial to your skin. You might like to invest in a sleep app to track your sleep quality – however, it is best to remove your phone from your room if you can.

2. How long you've been exposed to screens (your phone, TV, etc.). Why?

Believe it or not, while we're sitting in close proximity to screens on a daily basis, the blue light they emit has a negative impact on the skin. If you work at a computer, quit … I jest. (Humour will also be a recurring theme in this book.) In modern-day life, screens can't be avoided – if they can, that's impressive – so all I ask is that you're mindful of the time you spend in front of them and aim to cut down.

3. How much time you have spent in daylight. Why?

The body can produce Vitamin D through exposure to the sun, and Vitamin D affects your skin and your mental health in a positive way. So, we need daylight – but we need to seek it with caution (stay tuned).

4. How much 'me time' you've had. Why?

Time to destress and decompress will benefit your skin. This is important. I aim for thirty minutes of 'me time' a day. But sometimes, being busy, I might only manage 15. If you can't get it in one go, break it up into five minutes in the morning and five to ten minutes in the evening – you can incorporate your skincare routine into that 'me time'. Five minutes is better than no minutes. Driving, singing, walking, sitting and gymming all count. It doesn't have to be a spa day to be an investment in yourself.

Diet

5. How much sugar you've consumed. Why?

Refined sugar causes inflammation in the skin, which leads to a number of varying skin concerns. Stick to naturally occurring sugars in fruit instead. I appreciate sugar is addictive and delicious, but your skin is an organ!

6. How much water you're drinking. Why?

Water affects the internal moisture levels of your skin. You should drink one-and-a-half to two litres of water per day. Attempt to drink room temperature water as it is kinder to the gut, a key organ closely linked to the skin (as you'll soon learn). I am also a fan of eating your water – get it in via fruit and vegetables.

7. How much protein you've eaten. Why?

You are what you eat, so eat ingredients that will help you to make collagen. Protein is essential to boost collagen and elastin. I would advise you up your protein intake (just get more of it where possible) and ensure you are getting protein in at lunch and dinner – many people don't fancy protein first thing in the morning and that's OK, but remember, eggs are a great source of protein and perfect in the AM.

8. How many carbohydrate-rich foods you've eaten. Why?

Carbs are a key component in any healthy diet (which leads to good skin health), despite being seen by many dieters as the enemy. Get your carbs in via complex carbs (the good kind) which we'll explore more in the nutrition chapter. Unfortunately, that packet of crisps doesn't count as a good carb. Dam it.

9. How many good fats you've eaten. Why?

Good fats help to lubricate the skin - they are essentially an internal moisturiser. Again, try to incorporate good fats, such as fish, avocado, nuts, extra virgin olive oil and whole eggs, into your lunch and dinner.

10. How much caffeine you've consumed. Why?

Caffeine is a stimulant but can also trigger cortisol levels, which can exacerbate skin issues. But we want to be realistic when it comes to life changes – reduce your caffeine intake slowly rather than feel you have to stop now! If you drink four cups of caffeine per day, go down to three on week one, two the following week and aim to cope on one per day. We still need to enjoy vices in life, so there's no need to go completely caffeine free if you don't want to.

11. How much alcohol you've drunk. Why?

Alcohol leads to dreaded dehydration and you might even get good at spotting drinkles (dehydrated wrinkles). Again, I'm not going to tell you not to pop the prosecco to celebrate a life achievement but be aware of how your skin behaves after you have drunk alcohol. Does your skin suffer the following day? Is it red or tender or itchy? Dry? Spotty?

Yes, I know, that's a long list, but each and every one of the factors listed above pertains to your skin health.

If your skin is quite reactive, you may want to track the products you're using on it too, especially if you're introducing anything new. That way, you can separate the wheat from the chaff in your routine.

Why is your skin diary important?

If you're trying to get better skin and you're not seeing the results you want, a skin diary paints a very clear picture. If your skin is always dehydrated even though you're using products to combat this, it could actually be those two extras coffees per day or the lack of water that you're not thinking about. It may be a case that every third Wednesday of the month you get spots because of a stressful work meeting. This stress breakout can be prevented with proper nutrition in the week before.

The more we know, and the clearer the picture becomes, the more we can work on addressing our issues and concerns. And your diary will be most helpful in observing patterns if you fill it out over a three-month period (at least). For example, you may notice that your skin is oilier in week 1 and week 4 – and you can then look at the factors that may have caused this.

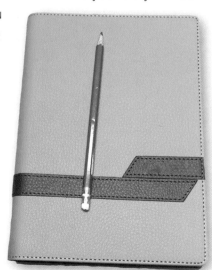

The skin diary concept will make more sense later on, especially when we cover the links between nutrition and skin, but it's imperative that you get started on this work now. You'll thank your future nerdie self.

Nerdie Tip: Don't forget Spritz O'Clock!

Please tick the box if:
- You have taken your vitamins and eaten clean **INSIDE**
- You applied your skincare regime **OUTSIDE**
- If applicable, you applied minimal makeup **ON TOP**
- Number of litres of **WATER** consumed

- Give yourself a number between 1-10 to reflect **STRESS** levels
- Was there more **SUGAR**?!
- Please list how many hours of **SLEEP** you had
- You have included **'ME TIME'** in your day
- Please list how many hours of **DAYLIGHT** you had

	Monday	Tuesday	Wednesday	Thursday	Friday	Saturday	Sunday
Inside							
Outside							
On Top							
Water							
Stress							
Sugar/ Diet							
Sleep							
'Me time'							
Daylight							
Additional comments							

Your Mindset

Before we get into the nitty-gritty of what makes your skin tick, we need to get ourselves on the same nerdie page.

In order to get the results you want, you need to get on board with not just the Skin Nerd philosophy, but the dos and don'ts of skincare, and adopt the right mental attitude. How you feel right now – your mindset – is your starting point on your skin-health journey. Not what you had for breakfast, not what serum you're massaging into your skin right this minute – your mindset. The rest will follow.

The Skin Nerd Philosophy

The skin is an organ and it should be respected accordingly. We poke and pick at our skin, we squeeze it like it's the end of a tube of toothpaste, we cover it in things that strip it dry and compromise its health. This is not right. The heart would not be disrespected in this way. We can see our skin, therefore we should shield it, feed it and respect it. It is not an accessory.

The 360° approach to skincare involves:

- Inside (nutrition, supplements, lifestyle)
- Outside (topical skincare, treatments)
- On top (SPF, makeup)

Looking at all these elements together, you get the whole picture. True skin health is like a jigsaw puzzle in that all the pieces need to fit together. No single part of the approach will deliver total skin health. It's a cumulative, holistic process.

Together we will cut through the marketing hype and assist in picking the right pieces and putting the puzzle together.

How Do You *Feel*?

The first question my team and I always ask a client at the outset of our work together is: 'How do you feel about your skin?'

It's heartbreaking to hear some of the answers from clients of all ages: 'I hate it', 'It gets me down every day', 'I won't leave the house if I am having a bad skin day', 'My mood is entirely dependent on how my skin is on a given day, which isn't ideal'. Men, you might be surprised to hear, often have the same response. The reality is, I can totally relate. Having bad skin is all encompassing. It's not a vanity issue. It's a health issue, and your feeling down about it is justified. It interrupts your daily musings, activities, plans and, ultimately, it chips away at your confidence.

I have real, unbridled empathy for those who struggle with their skin. I know first-hand how skin problems can affect your self-esteem and wellbeing. The condition of my skin has a massive impact on my mental health, my confidence and my mood. Every time I am run down or exhausted with stressful meetings to attend, spots creep out of my skin, like kids emerging at the sound of an ice-cream van's jingle. (In fact, even typing the word 'ice-cream', I swear new spots are forming – we'll get to the topic of sugar shortly.) Skin issues affect my confidence and for me, can be the difference between not looking people in the eye and holding my head high.

As The Skin Nerd, I am expected to have perfect skin. Unfortunately, because of systemic and genetic reasons, I do not. I'm not genetically predisposed to radiant, even and spot-free skin – I work for it just as you do (or just as you *will*). Just because I have the knowledge necessary to achieve good skin, and help others to too, doesn't mean I am immune from a breakout myself. And just as we get you to a point of clear, glowing skin, that doesn't mean you will never have another breakout or dry patch or phase of sensitivity at some point in your life. That isn't a promise I can make. Life gets in the way. Stress is unavoidable. But because I work with my skin every day, inside and out – treating it as part of my self-care routine – I can get pretty darn close. And because you'll do the work necessary, so will you.

Have you started that diary yet?

This confidence issue is why I do what I do, and it's a major goal of this book – to help you achieve not only healthy, glowing skin, but to regain your confidence and empower you to feel like the badass woman (or man) that you are.

I don't claim to be a psychologist but having an understanding of how our skin – good and bad – can impact on our mental health is very important. Unfortunately, marketing campaigns and social media don't always help matters. They can prey on our vulnerability and make us feel worse than we already do; our social feeds are filled with imagery of superhumans who are pore free, scar free and devoid of lines, and the subliminal pressure this puts us under is insane.

Those images are unrealistic (and, erm, photoshopped) and quite frankly boring. We don't walk around in real life with the Abu Dhabi filter in front of our face. So please know that, yes, your skin-health issues will have an impact on the way you feel but also be mindful of the fact that the content you consume can often exacerbate the issue. Take it all with a pinch of salt (but not too much salt because your skin won't like that either).

If things are sounding pretty bleak right now, worry not, we are only at the beginning of our journey together. Even just a few weeks into a skincare plan, we touch base with our clients again and ask them the same question: 'How do you feel now?' It's incredibly rewarding to hear people's responses:

'I actually feel good.'

'I feel better.'

'I will leave the house without makeup.'

'I've applied for the job I wanted.'

'I've gone on a date.'

The effects of their skincare plans go beyond what they see in the mirror and positively impact on all aspects of their lives.

Beyond Aesthetics

I have found that thinking about your skin's health and not just the way it looks helps when it comes to how you feel about your appearance aesthetically. Thinking about your skin's processes, which we'll tease apart, can shift your focus from how it looks to how amazing the skin is as an organ. There's a whole lot more than meets the eye and it's damn impressive. Do you ever take a moment to think about how your skin renews itself, protects everything inside you and keeps itself moisturised? Do you congratulate it daily as you wash it in the shower? It deserves a round of applause IMO. Respect that glorious organ.

In nailing your mindset, you also need to embrace the idea of consistency. What some clients are loathe to hear at the outset is that just as a single workout does not a toned physique make, the occasional skincare ritual does not achieve healthy skin. (I wish this wasn't the case too!) Consistency over time in your routine is what will get results. One night without using your Vitamin A serum, for example, is one less night it's not strengthening your skin's structure. But it gets easier and becomes habit. You will start to enjoy those few minutes in the morning and the same at night, knowing you are doing such good for your skin's health. If you work out regularly at the gym, you will see visible changes in your body over time. The same is true of your skin.

A Mindless Versus Mindful Approach to Skin Health

Here's what we're going to swap out right now: Ditch the mindless approach and choose the mindful approach to skin health.

A mindless approach to skin is following arbitrary guidelines that have been passed on to you through the media, through celebrities and public figures, and through marketing. Mindless skincare is all surface with little emphasis on nutrition and the reality of our daily lives.

On the other – far better – hand, a mindful approach means having and knowing the reason you have chosen every single product you use and working on long-term skin health rather than short-term results.

A mindful life is trying your best to be in tune with everything that happens in your body, in your mind and in your life. A mindful approach to skin is exactly the same: it's about considering the extrinsic and intrinsic factors affecting your skin, and putting certain things in motion to help with this. I have not always believed in a 360° approach to the skin. This idea was first introduced to me six years ago, and it was life-changing. Examining all aspects holistically is what makes the Nerdie approach mindful.

What Now?

Keep calm. If your skin is in the midst of a rough patch – or maybe there's something that's plagued you for years – this is what I want you to hear. I, of all people, know that there is nothing funny about breakouts, especially when they are recurrent and constant. But one thing is for certain when it comes to each individual breakout: it will come to an end. Whatever your skincare situation right now, it can and will improve. In fact, I'm 99 per cent certain that there is always a way to at least create a minimal change to even the most severe of concerns. Things will get better and things will fluctuate along the way. It might be a bumpy road (pun intended), especially in times of massive hormonal upheaval or emotional turmoil or when you're enjoying yourself to the fullest on a holiday where your main food group is gelato. But your skin today is not the skin you're stuck with. There is a light at the end of the tunnel.

Similarly, if you have good skin now, you need to maintain it.

By the end of this book, we will have achieved a new mindset. One that wakes up to a spot on your chin and says, 'OK, this is not ideal, but I know what I need to do to address this in the short term and in the long term.' You will be thoroughly educated and, remember, knowledge is always power. You will know your own skin and how it behaves, and you will be able to make better skincare choices.

Skin Diary Check-in:

Have a think about your mindset.

Note how you feel about your skin right now and outline your mindset for the days and weeks ahead.

Track your emotions as you go on this skin journey – both how you feel about your skin and how your general emotional state might be affecting your skin.

The Nerdie Principles

First things first. It's time to lay down the Skin Nerd laws – which I fondly refer to as the 10 Skin Nerd Commandments – and I advise strongly that you follow them. Why should I decree what you do with your skin? There are countless people and experts out there with varying opinions, and plenty of conflicting research would leave you with one massive headache. Everything I say throughout this book – and within these commandments – comes from working with many brands, philosophies and experts in the world.

I have ten years of trial and error behind me. I learn first-hand every day through speaking to clients and noting their feedback. Within our first year of business, we saw just shy of 5,000 hoomans. The results I see are what I go on. Embrace following the Skin Nerd Commandments, take the dos and don'ts on board and, with a little daily effort, the journey ahead will feel a lot less like climbing Mount Skinimanjaro and, instead, will be an idyllic learning experience with tangible and lasting results.

Return to these guidelines again and again to ensure they're permanently etched onto your brain.

The 10 Skin Nerd Commandments

1. Thou shalt aim for seven hours of restful sleep to maximise the skin's healing ability.

While you sleep, your skin is no longer busy trying to constantly protect you from everyday life. This means that it has proper time to heal and regenerate at night – immunity, metabolism and hydration levels have time to adapt and to regulate. Among many issues, not getting enough sleep can lead to fluid pooling under your skin, which is the puffiness that many people find under their eyes when they've under-slept.

PS. Napping doesn't count. The energy needed to repair the cells during sleep is being used elsewhere during daylight hours. Also having a high-quality sleep is essential: REM – rapid eye movement, the period of sleep when we dream – is a real concept not just a band (if you're familiar with the musicians I'm referring to you can skip straight to anti-ageing – just kidding, don't go anywhere right now). When you sleep, your blood flow increases so your skin refreshes itself, cells are given nutrients, your body relaxes into REM which enables it to re-energise and recuperate from the day that's just ended and prepare itself for the day that's about to start.

2. Thou shalt drink eight glasses of water daily to keep the skin hydrated and healthy.

Water hydrates the whole body, including the skin. You do, however, need to ensure that you're also consuming enough essential fatty acids to keep the water in (more on this later). While water alone is not the answer – nothing alone is the answer – it is needed for life and for us to perform optimally. Hydration is the key to skin volume. Up to 60 per cent of the adult human body is comprised of water as is the skin, and the more water the skin has, the plumper it appears and the more support it has.

If your skin is dehydrated, it will feel tight, taut and may have a coarse texture to it. Think of a raisin versus a grape – our goal is the juicy grape! Visually and aesthetically this means the skin has a childlike youthfulness and dewiness to it, with plenty of moisture to boot.

3. Thou shalt avoid processed food.

I know – this one is difficult to maintain at all times, but processed foods affect the body and the skin's immunity. They are full of empty calories and empty in skin value too, so try at the very least to reduce your intake. Processed foods are dosed in preservatives and salt that can affect immunity. They also affect your lymphatic system as these kinds of food take more effort to drain and waste, which, in turn, causes inflammation, which includes redness, ageing, spots, psoriasis and eczema.

4. Thou shalt keep sugar intake low.

I've a lot to say about sugar but, for now, know that the sweet stuff also causes inflammation (the body's way of fighting something that it perceives as a threat, such as infection), which is usually associated with redness, swelling, heat or pain. It also speeds up the ageing process as well as reducing the skin's immunity. When my clients reduce their sugar intake, their skin congestion, which includes spots, blackheads and clogged pores is often halved, with redness considerably reduced after some months.

5. Thou shalt eat lots of vegetables.

When your mother force fed you broccoli as a kid, she was right. We need to eat vegetables to feed the skin from within with potent antioxidants that control the rate at which we age. Antioxidants are the unsung heroes of skin health — they literally armour your skin against the environment. An antioxidant is essentially a cell's defence force that fights against nasties, such as stress, excess UV exposure, excess alcohol consumption and smoking.

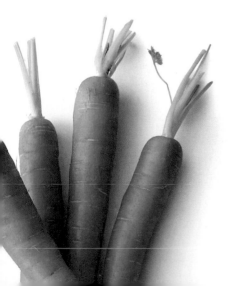
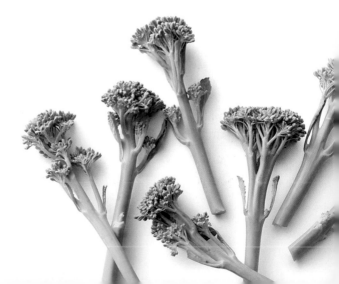

6. Thou shalt consume adequate amounts of protein.

Protein isn't just for those gym gains, it helps to boost collagen in the body. Collagen is a protein found in the lower layer if the skin – a layer far beyond what we can see and touch – and is responsible for the structure of the skin and the 'bounce' associated with the skin's youthful appearance. It is also responsible for lining capillary walls and the skin's ability to heal from things such as stretch marks. Our naturally created levels of collagen and elastin tend to diminish after we turn twenty-five. (Most skincare brands say that forty is the age at which you should get on the anti-ageing buzz. Wrong.) We should start to introduce more protein into our diets at this early stage. Make sure you're getting your protein at lunch and dinner every day. The recommended amount is 0.8 grams per kilogram of body weight.

7. Thou shalt gobble up good fats.

Good fats, such as those found in avocados, are the key ingredient for locking in skin hydration, reducing irritation and reactive skin conditions. They lock in goodness. The word 'fat' is often feared when, in fact, it is a keyword and ingredient for skin health. Fat, more specifically essential fatty acids, is key for conditions such as eczema, psoriasis and acne-prone skin, because the fat will act as an anti-inflammatory agent and an internal moisturiser. You're looking for monounsaturated fats, such as Omega 6, found in nuts, seeds and fish.

Bad fats are trans fats (trans fatty acids). They are synthetic or artificially produced and you'll often find 'hydrogenated' in the ingredients of the products that contain it.

8. Thou shalt reduce your caffeine intake.

Caffeine increases stress levels, particularly the production of the stress hormone cortisol. Heightened stress worsens chronic skin conditions and causes dehydration of the skin. Caffeine is something we all gravitate towards – I'd be lying if I said I didn't enjoy a cup of tea as much as the next person – but for optimal skin health, reduce your consumption over time to one cup per day.

9. Thou shalt not smoke.

This one's obviously a no-no for countless well-documented reasons but the cigarettes you puff on in the smoking area also decrease the flow of oxygen to your skin (affecting its tone and pallor) while robbing your body of Vitamin C, which is an essential nutrient to synthesise (the nerdie word for 'create more') collagen. And, no, smoking is not something you can just 'reduce', this is something you need to kick in the proverbials right now. Non-negotiable. Sorry, not sorry!

10. Thou shalt exercise.

Ensure you exercise regularly not just to promote health, but so that your cardio-vascular system can assist with lymphatic draining. Weight training tones the muscle which lies under the skin and so enables the skin to appear firmer and more taut. It also stimulates blood flow to give your skin the highly coveted glow. Be careful to cleanse thoroughly after exercise though, to make sure the sudoriferous glands (nerd name for 'sweat glands') don't get clogged.

Skin Sins:

1. **DON'T** EVER use facial wipes. 'But?' I hear you cry, 'But what if?' NOPE. Do not even get me started. They cause   irritation and sensitivity over prolonged periods of use.

2. **DON'T** over-expose yourself to UV rays. Whether it is through sunbed usage or simply not wearing your sunscreen, over-exposing your skin to UV rays is a cardinal Skin Sin. Apply SPF all year around. Protect and repair is key. Protect that wonderful organ and give it a helping hand in blocking the pollution and harmful sun rays.

    Using sunbeds is irresponsible and dangerous. If you use them, stop it. Now!

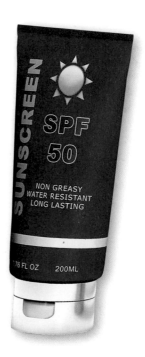

3. **DON'T** ignore the importance of your diet.

4. **DON'T** buy products based on their pretty packaging and sexy scents and expect results. Smells do not change cells®. In fact, perfumed products can irritate your skin So, as a rule of thumb, never choose a product based on its scent. That's what candles and perfume are for, OK? And while I'm at it, the same goes for pretty packaging. Going forwards, you will be able to use the knowledge in this book when buying products and will become a skin nerd yourself.

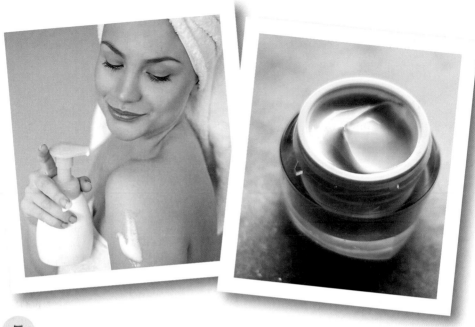

5. **DON'T** believe in mass-marketing campaigns based on hype alone. Some big brands spend more money on marketing than on the product research and development. This isn't reassuring. An expensive product isn't necessarily better than a cheaper one – it's all about the skingredients.

6. **DON'T** buy a product because a celebrity adores it unless you know it will suit your skin.

7. **DON'T** self-diagnose. A good consultation with an expert is essential and this is why I've created my online consultancy business. It's so important for me to analyse someone's skin (which we do online) to be able to give them the most specific and personal advice possible. Align yourself with someone you trust completely.

8. **DON'T** view skin treatments as a once-a-year treat – they need to mirror a good skin regime at home.

9. **DON'T** obsess over your skin (as hard as I know this is). This gets nobody anywhere except further into the depths of despair and stress and will only hold you back.

10. Last, but by no means least, **DON'T** forget that the skin is an organ.

Sounds like there's very little room for fun here, doesn't it? Skin is serious. In the same way good fats are bossy boots that keep hydration in your skin, you have to be a bossy boots to yourself sometimes too. Why? Because you care.

Look. We are all hooman – myself included – and I have a sweet tooth and I like to enjoy myself. The main thing is to understand how something like a big gloopy sticky fudgy ice-cream sundae affects your skin. It will be much easier to cope with a bad skin day if you fully understand how and why it's happened, as well as how to rectify it. Ignorance is not bliss in the skincare scenario if you want real results.

Ultimately, though, we have to let our hair down from time to time.

In relation to all the above – aside from wipes and cigarettes and sunbeds which are definite no-nos – start with small changes. Small changes make a big difference.

And now, assuming we're all on the very

same page, we move forward towards understanding the skin anatomy. Notebooks at the ready!

Skin Diary Check-in:

Write out the skin commandments and sins most relevant to your situation right now.

Create a timeline and checklist for yourself – for example, 'I will reduce my coffee intake to two cups a day.' Set a reminder in your phone for two weeks' time. Chances are you will have slipped back into bad habits, so this will help you get back on track.

Skin Anatomy

With The Skin Nerd philosophy forever ingrained on your grey matter, we can now get down to the nitty-gritty of skin. My guilty pleasure.

Brace yourself for some hardcore science here, but, worry not, I'll explain everything as simply as I can and I won't be testing you on your skin science vocabulary. At the very least you'll sound impressive at your next dinner party (you can check out the nerdie glossary if you need a refresher).

The thing is, it can be difficult to visualise what exactly your skincare is doing if you have no idea what the physiological makeup of your skin is. Knowing how your skin is structured, and what it needs, helps you to reimagine it as an organ rather than a sheath draped across everything else in your body – and this will help you better understand how you can help it out. When you get this, everything that comes after only takes a little bit of 'skinformed' effort.

Before we tease apart the various layers of our skin (figuratively not literally), let's consider the role of our skin as a whole.

What Is the Role of the Skin?

The role of our skin is complex and noble. As I've mentioned before, people sometimes forget that that their skin isn't purely aesthetic – it's actually the largest organ of the body. The skin is made up of a group of tissues that, together, form our most powerful protective layer, defending our bodies against the things that we don't want anywhere near our insides.

The skin's job is to protect us. It shields us from the environment. It keeps the good in and the bad out. Among its many functions, it's responsible for the secretion of oils (e.g. the oil that lubricates the hair follicles and moisturises the skin) and the absorption of what we need (e.g. Vitamin A), enabling active ingredients to penetrate. It's also our hero when it comes to heat regulation, keeping our internal temperature at 38° Celsius.

Within the skin, there are three key layers: the epidermis, the dermis and the hypodermis.

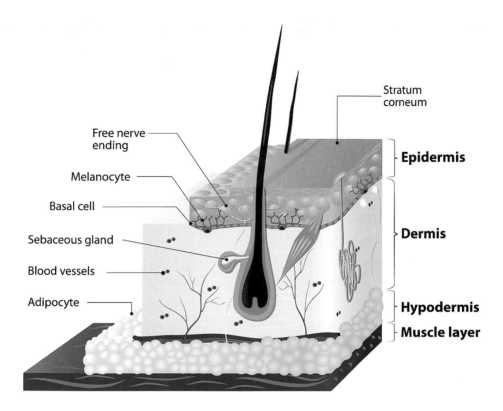

Labels on figure:
- Stratum corneum
- Free nerve ending
- Melanocyte
- Basal cell
- Sebaceous gland
- Blood vessels
- Adipocyte
- Epidermis
- Dermis
- Hypodermis
- Muscle layer

The Epidermis

The epidermis varies in depth, depending on the part of the body you're looking at – for example, the soles of the feet are the thickest while the eyelids and your nipples are the thinnest.

- The top sublayer of the epidermis is the *stratum corneum*. This skin layer is constantly shedding, and constantly trying to renew itself. In fact, it's suggested that most of your house dust is made up of skin cells. Sexy, eh? If it wasn't enough to have a good skincare routine, you also have to vacuum yourself up weekly.

- Under the *stratum corneum*, you'll find the *stratum lucidum*. However, this second layer is only found under the soles of the feet and palms of the hands, so it isn't always mentioned – but I want to give you the full picture.

- For everywhere else on the body, you'll find the *stratum granulosum* under the *stratum corneum*. The *stratum granulosum* acts as a barrier between the *stratum corneum* and the *stratum spinosum* and prevents unwanted chemicals and debris from getting any further into your body.

- Then you have the *stratum spinosum*, otherwise known as the 'prickly cell layer'. The cells in this layer contain cell structures that help with binding the cells to each other. It is in this binding process that the cells become 'prickly' in shape (with little spiny projections) because of the structures that have caused the binding.

- The base layer of the epidermis is known as the *stratum germinativum*. This is where skin cells are made in a process called mitosis. This layer will dictate the health of the skin cell being made. The more healthy it is , the more healthy the cells being made will be. It's also where you'll find pigment, the melanin granules created by our melanocyte cells (the pigment-making cell) that protects us from UV damage and gives us our genetic colour.

The 'Mother Cell'

The keratinocyte cell is the type of cell that makes up around 90 per cent of the epidermis. Keratinocyte cells in the basal layer (*stratum germinativum*) – which are known as 'basal cells'– are the cells that divide to create new ones (via mitosis). They are also known as 'mother cells' because they are literally the mothers of other new cells. If the DNA of these cells is damaged by life and lifestyle (pollution, smoking, alcohol, etc.), the cells that they go on to create are not as healthy as they should be. This creates something of a vicious circle – unhealthy skin creates more unhealthy skin.

The Dermis

This is the true living layer of the skin and is just below the epidermis. In it, you find components such as collagen and elastin, blood vessels, hair follicles and sweat glands. This is also the layer of skin where change can occur, even though most of the products we buy in supermarkets only sit on top of the epidermis. For example, moisturisers that feel luxurious to the touch may make an instant impact on how our skin feels, but they do not go any deeper than the *stratum corneum*. This is not to say these kinds of products are bad, but, if we want to create real change, we need the kinds of products you'd usually obtain via a professional consultation – ones which contain active ingredients. These products reach the lower layer of the epidermis and can send messages into the dermis to trigger collagen and elastin production.

The dermis is composed of its own set of sublayers, but there are just two: the papillary dermis and the reticular dermis. Yes, more extras from *Jurassic Park*.

- The papillary dermis is made up of white collagen fibres and yellow elastic fibres (mainly elastin), which are the two anti-ageing proteins. These are what make your skin look plump and enable it to adhere to the contours of your body, which is why our skin sags as we age.

- The reticular dermis is underneath the papillary dermis, and comprises blood vessels, lymph vessels, nerve endings, sweat glands and their ducts, hairs and sebaceous (oil) glands.

Our blood vessels supply each and every cell and structure in the dermis with oxygen and nutrients, helping to feed everything that creates a healthy skin cell. When these capillaries (small blood vessels) weaken or collapse, we see the appearance of broken capillaries on the surface of the skin (fine red lines that look like veins). This is just one reason why we need Vitamin C as it strengthens the capillary walls within the dermis.

Our lymph vessels gather interstitial fluid (the fluid that tissue cells bathe in) and deliver it to the bloodstream.

Our nerve endings let us know there is pain occurring. Our sweat glands help us to regulate body temperature and help to provide the skin with natural moisturising factors.

Our hairs help to direct oil towards the surface of the skin so that it is hydrated and moisturised, while our sebaceous glands secrete sebum into hair follicles (which you'll find everywhere except the palms of your hands and the soles of your feet). Sebum prevents the skin from becoming infected. It also waterproofs the skin and stops it from drying out. Sebum is often perceived as the 'baddy'. It is not!

Hypodermis

Beneath *these* two crucial layers you'll find the hypodermis – also known as subcutaneous tissue.

The hypodermis contains cells that create connective tissues and produce the protein necessary to connect the epidermis to the dermis. The hypodermis insulates us – it's our protective shell, like a fiberglass coat – and its fat cells are storage units for energy and nutrients.

So that's a brief look at how our skin is structured (you may need a quick breather but this diagram should help).

How Does the Skin Function?

Our skin cells have a special gene known as the 'clock gene' that is linked to our circadian rhythm, which is also known as your 'sleep/wake cycle'. Our skin functions in tandem with our circadian rhythm to set out when the skin goes into different phases of repair.

The skin repairs its DNA at times when there is less likely to be UV exposure, such as in the evening. It's also carrying out its role as protector during the day and is continuously fending off possible damage. At night, new skin cells are created. This is when our blood circulation improves, and oxygen and nutrients are delivered to the skin cells.

Night-time is crucial for skin as this is when it repairs, tackling any damage that has occurred throughout the day. Skin cell proliferation (your skin's natural exfoliation process) happens at night and this is why your skin may look fabulous when you wake up but not as bright, clean or as fresh a few hours into the day.

How Your Skin Functions with Products

The purpose of skincare products is to assist your skin to carry out its processes to the best of its ability. What you put on your skin is merely an aid to what it already does, or what it used to be able to do but struggles with because of ageing. To give a helpful analogy, when you're using the right skingredients, your skin benefits – like the benefits someone feels who has been jogging for six months rather than someone who has been jogging for a day. At six months, your body finds it easier to run than it did on day one.

In the same way, products do a lot of the work for your skin. Products, when appropriate, keep your skin fit. For example, products rich in antioxidants help your skin battle free-radical damage, while sunscreen works to shield it from UV rays so that it doesn't need to try as hard to fend from them itself.

The Skin Cycle

In beauty advertising and marketing, you'll hear a lot about cell regeneration or the skin cycle. But what exactly is this and how long does it take our skin cells to regenerate?

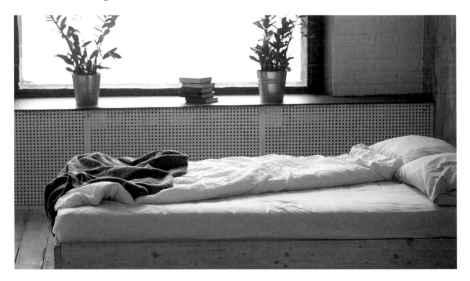

I like to use a bed analogy when it comes to the cell turnover process:

- The base of the bed is like the hypodermis (i.e. the storage or base).

- The mattress is the dermis (i.e the main bulk of the structure that can dip and pucker if springs (elastin) are broken).

- The sheets are the top layers we can touch (i.e. the *stratum corneum*).

The mattress (dermis) affects how seamless the sheets (skin we can see) appears. It's all from the inside out.

Skin cells are made in the bottom layer of the epidermis, the aforementioned *stratum germinativum*. Then, they all head on a journey to the top where they are sloughed off via the skin's natural exfoliation process.

In a healthy skin cell, this skin cycle takes about twenty-eight days – let's call it a month. Our rate of skin cell regeneration slows down as we get older, hence our skin can become duller in appearance as we age. In the case of acne or congested, sluggish-looking skin, the cycle is longer and is often characterised by the density of the *stratum corneum* (the top layer that we can touch). On the extreme end of the scale, a client who suffers with psoriasis will have a rapid skin cell turnover, so this cycle happens too fast.

Extrinsic and Intrinsic Factors that Affect Skin

It's time now to explore all the factors that have an impact on your skin. To make this as clear as possible, I have divided these factors into two different categories: extrinsic and intrinsic.

Intrinsic factors

Intrinsic, for the most part, refers to genetics or things that happen inside your body. These factors are sometimes beyond your control, such as hormone levels or medical conditions. All these things impact your skin.

Genes

Genetic factors are anything that has been passed down through your family line, a bit like an heirloom.

The things we inherit include skin types, skin conditions and the rate at which we age. But if you've inherited certain negative issues, this is not a life sentence. We can work with your genetics. Similarly, if your parents had great skin, this does not mean you can throw in the towel and guzzle the Peanut M&Ms. Good genes are not a golden ticket.

Whatever your genes, you can leave things as they are – but this is not a great idea. You have to work with your genetics to give yourself the best chance of healthy skin. For example, if you come from a long line of people with accelerated ageing, you need to be more conscious of prevention. In that same sense, those who are genetically predisposed to great skin with no issues whatsoever assume that they don't need to use sunscreen because they don't visibly burn. People who wash their faces with a bar of soap and use products without much consideration, may wonder why their skin isn't in the best condition later in life.

Whatever your genetic predisposition, nobody is born well-protected from UVA rays and no matter how long you've used soap for, it doesn't mean it suits your skin. Nobody comes out of the womb with a pollution shield on them either – you still need to be using antioxidants. You need to invest in your skin regardless of genetics.

Hormones and stress

'Hormones' and 'stress' are two words that get thrown about a lot in skincare. In my opinion, there is a lot of confusion about them, with hormones given far too much weight when, in reality, it's often stress that causes many of the hormonal changes that lead to skin issues. When it comes to hormones, there are some issues you won't be able to control or will need medication to control (it might be best to consult a GP to get a better understanding of what might be happening in your body if you suspect a hormonal issue), but there are some factors you can control, such as the impact of a high-sugar diet on your hormone levels. If we ease off the sugar, we calm down the hormones involved.

Ideally, what you're looking for is 'homeostasis'. This is when all your hormones are in harmony with one another, when everything is balanced. A hormonal balance is an intrinsic factor, but when the hormonal imbalance is brought about by diet or stress, it becomes an extrinsic factor, which is more to do with our lifestyle. I know, it's a little confusing at first, but bear with me.

Stress is often a major culprit behind a lack of homeostasis and while it can be caused by things outside the body – which we can work to improve – the effects of stress are often felt inside the body, or on the skin. Stress affects the skin in several ways.

One is an increase in cortisol levels. A sudden surge in cortisol, caused by something outside of the body, can affect your immune system, causing inflammation that can contribute to poor skin health. A spike in cortisol can also trigger further flare-ups of psoriasis or eczema or rosacea for those who struggle with these conditions. Ask anyone who suffers from one of these skin conditions and you can bet your bottom dollar they will say it's worse during stressful times.

The reason for the flood of cortisol is because your body is preparing you to be able to cope with a threat from the outside. However, your mind and body can't tell the difference between a stressful exam, a meeting with your boss or a literal threat to your safety.

Another effect of stress is that it drives up another type of hormone called androgens, a male sex hormone. Androgens are supposed to control sebum production but when they're in excess, they stimulate oil glands, leading to extra oil being produced and thus more blackheads (trapped oil), papules (spots without the bacteria whiteheads) and pustules (spots with bacteria whitehead) forming on the skin.

The effects of stress are felt inside your body, and, for some people, the effects can manifest on their skin. Stress is often the result of issues in your work life or your personal life or other things that are simply outside of your control.

Stress can also stop you from getting enough sleep, leading to puffy eyes and dark circles, and, as we explore next, it can affect your gut too by disrupting the delicate balance of good bacteria, thus triggering skin problems. On top of this, stress creates lines that you can see almost immediately (don't tell me you don't furrow your brow when you're stressed). All in all, stress is nobody's friend.

What's more, stressing about the effects of stress on your skin only adds to the problem. It becomes a vicious cycle because stressing about your skin may worsen it and the worsening of your skin will increase your stress levels. Because of all of this, stress management is crucial when it comes to getting your skin to a healthy place. Rather than solely attacking the skin concern, or that one spot on your chin, you need to target the stress itself. We pull weeds by the roots, don't we?

I like to factor in plenty of 'me time' to bring myself back to centre and quell my stress levels (remember, those 15 minutes a day, at least, are the goal). I will regularly opt for a walk on the beach. I also incorporate mindfulness into my daily skincare routine, breathing deeply for the few minutes it takes both morning and night – or at traffic lights, or at regular intervals in between. Breathing: so simple, so key.

Periods

Now let's talk about periods, another intrinsic factor. Periods are a cyclical event similar to our skin cycle. Every woman's period is different, but here's how the skin functions, generally speaking, around menstruation.

In the few days preceding your period, your progesterone levels rise, so your sebaceous glands produce more sebum. A spike in progesterone can lead to pores that are more closed and this, in turn, means that debris and dead skin cells will find it harder to escape the pore, leading to them becoming trapped and, so, spots form.

Given that P. acnes (part of our skin's acid mantle, short for propioni-bacterium acnes, a bacteria that lives on the skin) loves sebum so much, you'll see more of this clingy bacteria too, leading to more inflamed spots.

At the end of your period, your progesterone levels will drop drastically and so will your skin's production of sebum and oils, which is why some people get dryness around this time. However, your oestrogen levels will rise, so your skin should appear fresh and clear outside of possible dryness as your production of collagen will increase.

Gut health

Another intrinsic factor that you need to be mindful of is your gut. We say the skin is a barometer for your internal health; well your gut is also a reliable indicator of your health in general. A healthy gut doesn't just mean no tummy issues, it also means healthier skin. Don't be dubious. I have observed this reality in thousands of my clients.

Here's how it works in relation to skin: we absorb skin-loving nutrients through the small intestine, which isn't really small at all. We need to absorb as much as possible, which is why we should chew food thoroughly so that it becomes absorbable. The stomach digests proteins through the work of digestive enzymes, which we can boost by taking supplements, (something I do myself). We need proteins for our whole body to be healthy so that our skin can function optimally.

Our gut, just like our skin, has its own ecosystem of bacteria. An overgrowth of bacteria means that the excess bacteria can steal nutrients from us, and an imbalance in bacteria in our gut can mean poor digestion. Because of this, I believe probiotics (yeasts and live bacteria) are essential to skin health. They improve our general health and this, in turn, has a positive effect on the skin. My skin's healing ability, clarity and tone is greatly improved when I am taking probiotic supplements and digestive enzyme supplements.

The gut–skin axis is the phrase often used to describe the interaction between the gut and the skin and the subsequent consequences of this interaction. Links have been found between inflammatory bowel diseases and inflammatory skin diseases, and, in studies done by the Korean Academy of Asthma, Allergy and Clinical Immunology and the University of Genoa, it was shown that those with rosacea were more likely to also have small intestine bacterial overgrowth.

When we are stressed, we tend not to absorb our food quite as well because our bodies go into fight-or-flight mode. When this happens, our digestive system can slow down or even shut down entirely. Our bodies think we are in danger (stress), so they shut down any system that isn't necessary for our survival. Instead, we'll have increased heart rates (so we can run away), and other stress symptoms. When this happens, we're no longer absorbing that goodness from our gut, which means our skin is also not getting what it needs. By now, you should be starting to understand the ecosystem of your whole body. Everything works together but factors, such as stress, can throw that harmony off. Again, our goal is to restore homeostasis.

Gut health remains an intrinsic factor for those with gut conditions, but, as our gut health is largely determined by our lifestyle this can also be considered an extrinsic factor; something you can very much control. For this reason, I would say gut health is both an intrinsic and extrinsic factor in one.

Extrinsic factors

Extrinsic factors are things within our environment that affect our general health and our skin health. These are the lifestyle choices that we make that impact on our skin.

What follows is a list of potential extrinsic factors in your life:
- smoking
- sugar intakc

- medication
- drinking alcoholic or sugary drinks
- eating processed food
- sleep (or a lack thereof)
- stress
- over-exercising
- pollution
- drinking water quality (limescale)
- the sun's UVA and UVB rays

Though you might not think it – and I know that when it comes to addictions like smoking it's easier said than done – the truth is that we can control the vast majority of these extrinsic lifestyle factors.

You are the driver of your life, nobody else is going to take the wheel. Why wait until Monday? If you want to prioritise it, you'll want to start now. If you value yourself, and value your skin as an organ, you will find the necessary self-motivation.

You *can* reduce sugar.

You *can* strive for balance.

You *can* make efforts to manage your stress on a daily basis and incorporate mindful breathing into your day.

You *can* protect from pollution-related damage by using antioxidants. If you believe your water quality is affecting your skin, filter it.

All these changes can be made before we even get on to the subjects of topical products and professional treatments. You can get yourself surprisingly close to full skin health by the actions you take.

Oxidation and Free Radicals

What is oxidation?

In our nerdie world, we talk a lot about oxidation. Even if you don't know it, you'll already be familiar with the concept – if you leave an apple exposed after biting it, the air oxidises the flesh of the apple and turns it brown, which means you have accelerated the amount of oxygen that got onto one area of the apple at one time and it has caused free-radical damage.

We need oxygen to survive. Every living cell needs oxygen to produce energy and build proteins, and oxygen provides our skin with nutrients – hence the popularity of oxygen masks in treatments. But too much oxygen at any one time can be counterproductive, because oxygen is one of the most unstable molecules we have on this planet. However, this instability is only an issue when it comes to our skin where it causes wear and tear, resulting in the accelerated ageing of skin cells.

Oxidation damages the DNA of the keratinocyte 'mother' cell, which causes further damage to the cell membrane and to the DNA of the nucleus, and this leads to the cell becoming reprogrammed and no longer as healthy as it once was. When oxidation occurs, the skin's healing ability becomes more sluggish. The skin is no longer functioning as it was designed to, and this opens you up to all manner of skin concerns, including being more prone to sensitisation or photodamage (light damage from daylight and heated ray light).

Oxidation in our daily life is caused by extrinsic factors, such as smoking, drinking alcohol, unrestful sleep and pollution. It also happens within us during cell turnover, which is something we cannot control ourselves. Oxidation is something that's going to happen regardless, but we can ease the process with antioxidants.

What are free radicals?

Simply put, a free radical is a by-product of oxidation. As we take in and use oxygen, we naturally create free radicals as a sort of waste product. These free radicals can then damage cells, proteins and DNA.

A free radical is an atom or molecule that has an unpaired electron (electrons like to travel in pairs, you see). This makes it unstable and it will do anything to stabilise itself.

You know when you have had a tough day at work and you practically run from the office to get home, diving on some chocolate and red wine? This is how free radicals feel. However, free radicals can't get their hands on a nice glass of Merlot inside your skin, so they try to pair their extra electron with a nearby healthier cell. This means that the other nearby cell becomes unstable too. So you have yet another free radical. This chain reaction continues within the skin causing minor destruction. This is why we don't like free radicals.

When there are masses of free radicals, they cause something known as oxidative stress, when there aren't enough antioxidants to settle the free radicals. Oxidative stress is what causes damage to cellular structures within the skin, whether they be fat cells, DNA or the skin's proteins (collagen and elastin). Over time, this causes your collagen and elastin to become damaged and depleted, which leads to crepe paper-like skin, laxity and ridging.

When your skin cells are damaged, you are also more susceptible to many skin conditions. For example, if you smoke, which is an activity that causes oxidation, you release a trillion free radicals into your body that attempt to attach themselves to a healthy cell to balance themselves on something secure – and, yep, that happens with every cigarette you smoke.

Antioxidants

What can we do about oxidation and free radicals? In a word – antioxidants, and the word itself explains what they do: fight oxidants.

Now, it should be known that we can't really stop oxidative stressors, such as light and pollution, from occurring and having negative effects on the skin, but we can limit the damage and the severity of the process with antioxidants as they neutralise the effects internally by balancing those spare electrons.

Often underestimated within the skindustry, antioxidants are a slow burner that we use to protect the skin long term. We will not see results immediately – as we would with many other products – and this is why they can often be overlooked. To show the effectiveness of antioxidants, we would need to examine the same person with the same lifestyle in two alternate universes, where one of them uses antioxidant protection and the other one doesn't. So you'll just have to take my word for it.

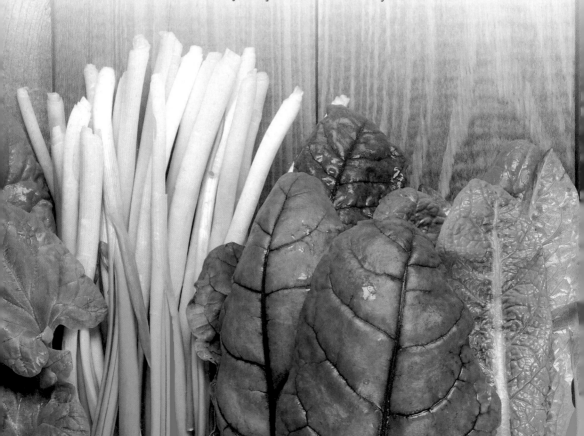

Going back to the apple analogy for a moment – if you squeeze lemon juice on an exposed apple, it will stop it from turning brown. This is how antioxidants work. They stop oxidation by balancing out the electron within the skin so the free radical does not need to attach itself to anything. They protect!

Antioxidants stop the chain reaction of free radicals by donating an electron to a free radical without turning into a free radical itself. Life is a free-radical exposure site and antioxidants are your protective armour. Antioxidants also protect against inflammation, which is at the root of many skin concerns.

You can fight against oxidation with antioxidants in two ways: internally with nutrition and externally with products. The exchange happens inside the skin, so we want to neutralise it as much as possible internally with a leafy green diet and plenty of antioxidant-rich fruit and vegetables (green tea also helps).

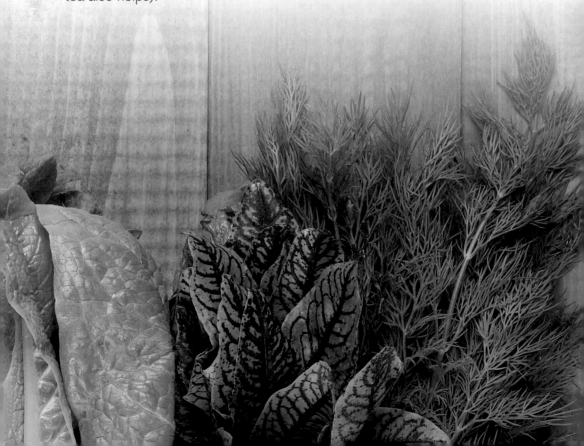

Imagine there is a crack in the foundation of a building and you're busy trying to fix the roof. On the outside, your skin is exposed to the elements, and pollution can collect on the surface of your skin. Here, we're guarding the free radicals from even getting onto the skin, so we are strengthening our skin's natural defence mechanism from both perspectives.

And that wraps up our overview of the skin and its anatomy.

Consider yourself skinformed.

Skin Diary Check-in:

List the intrinsic and extrinsic factors that may be influencing your skin concerns.

Think about:
- *What in your daily routine can you identify as an extrinsic factor?*
- *Could breakouts be coinciding with particularly stressful times at work?*
- *How has your digestion been?*
- *Is your gut health compromised and therefore affecting your skin?*

Nutrition

After reading this chapter, you'll understand why 'feed the skin from within' is my most overused phrase.

Treating the skin externally is one thing but it's not enough. For lasting results, we need to go back to our 360° perspective, and nutrition is a major, *major* factor in this approach. Treating your skin with products alone is like putting water on a fire while the gas is still turned on. For example, a cleanser will mop up excess oil but it is a short-term solution if used alone. If, however, we regulate our insides with nutrition, that will dictate how much oil we secrete externally.

Treating your skin internally gives you a second, more reliable layer of defence. Nutrients are carried throughout the bloodstream to feed your dermis (the deeper layer), where the connective tissues are and where proteins break down.

As I mentioned in the intro, no topical skincare can reach the dermis on its own. Many products claim to trigger activities within it, but the power to reach it lies within nutrition.

Before we look at the foods that you should be consuming for healthy skin, as well as the supplements that can help you along the way, I'm going to talk about some of the main offenders within our diets when it comes to poor skin health: sugar, dairy, alcohol and processed foods.

The Sunflower Analogy

For every consultation that I do, I show my client our pretty desk sunflowers. Everyone loves the top of the sunflower – it's yellow, appealing and vibrant. I touch the petals and say these represent the skin that we can touch and see. When you're planting the sunflower, you take time to consider the spacing between the sunflowers and the soil you're choosing to plant it in (with plenty of nutrients in it). You water from the root because you know it needs to be hydrated from the inside out. Imagine you witnessed me 'watering' the sunflower by just wetting the yellow petals. You'd decide there was little hope for the flower! You can't see goodness in the soil and at the roots, but having made the effort, you will have a beautiful, healthy flower. It's the same with your skin; the lower layers feed the layer above. If we rely solely on topical products, we are not truly feeding the skin where it is formed. And how you feed it from within will determine its health and appearance on the surface.

Sugar

First things first – sugar. One of the main offenders on our quest for skin health.

'What's the big deal with sugar and skin?' I hear you ask.

How long have you got?

For starters, it's worth understanding that sugars are converted into glucose in the body. Glucose raises insulin levels, which triggers inflammation, and this, over time, damages your collagen and elastin in your skin, leading to accelerated ageing. The joy! Please note that while ageing is a gift, accelerated ageing is self-inflicted.

When our collagen and elastin begin to degrade, our skin loses its elasticity and becomes less structured because it is these proteins that give it structure in the first place. These proteins are particularly susceptible to sugar damage. What's more, the inflammation affects the skin's healing ability. Across many of my clients who appear to be ageing beyond their years, even though they are not smoking and eating what they *think* is a healthy balanced diet, the common denominator is often sugar.

Sugar causes the formation of something known in my nerdie world as Advanced Glycation End products. Isn't it ironic that the acronym spells AGE? What are these obscure sounding things you ask? AGEs are sugar complexes created when the sugars that have been left unchecked in the bloodstream grab on to protein molecules (collagen and elastin) because they have to go somewhere. When this happens, the collagen and elastin become rigid (they are normally soft and supple) and can no longer do the heavy lifting for your skin. AGEs can trigger inflammation, which causes further tissue damage and accelerated ageing. What's more, the glycation process may also exacerbate existing skin conditions, such as rosacea or acne. How will you know you have AGEs? Are you prepared to grab a mirror or relative? Sugaring is often characterised within the skin as crisscross lines and wrinkles, like a hashtag #. Apart from premature ageing, in my experience, sugar can lead to a spike in androgens, which will increase your likelihood of breakouts.

More research is needed to confirm this as not everyone with a high sugar diet will have spots, but a 2002 study published in *Archives of Dermatology* shows strong evidence that acne is primarily a 'Western' disease. Researchers studied 1,200 people in Papua New Guinea and 115 people in Eastern Paraguay, where people eat fresh plant foods and lean meat they raise themselves, and they didn't see a single pimple. If sugar is what's missing from their diets, that can't just be a coincidence, right?

If all of that wasn't enough, the more sugar you eat, the more your insulin levels rise and, eventually, you develop insulin resistance which can manifest as excess hair growth (and we do not need to add a beard to the equation here) and discolouration of the skin. Insulin resistance also precedes the development of Type 2 diabetes.

Before you step away from the Dib Dab, we must be clear: when I say 'sugar', I don't just mean the Terry's Chocolate Orange sitting on your desk. Unfortunately, sugar is found in almost everything, but it's the sugar in simple carbohydrates that are the real problem – this includes foods such as white bread, white pasta, fruit juice and most sweet things.

And why are they the problem?

Because when these foods convert to glucose, which they do at lightning speed, they cause a spike in insulin, which leads to inflammation. (And, as mentioned earlier, inflammation is key to many conditions.)

This is why you'll hear more about the glycaemic index (GI) of foods these days. The GI scale determines how quickly blood sugar levels rise after eating a particular food. Certain foods, such as simple carbohydrates, have a high glycaemic index, which means they convert to sugar in the body rapidly. Foods with a low glycaemic index, such as green vegetables and brown rice, won't cause the same spike in insulin levels as they are broken down into glucose at a much slower rate. These low-GI foods delay sugar absorption and so they're better for your skin.

These foods still have sugar in them, but they are described as complex carbohydrates and they keep your sugar levels on an even keel, and so are much kinder to your skin.

When it comes to sugar, understanding the glycaemic index will help you to make better, more skin-friendly decisions.

The Glycaemic Index Scale 👓

The GI ranks foods from 1 to 100. The number a food is given explains how quickly that food is broken down when digested and transformed into a basic glucose. 100 represents pure glucose – so the higher the number, the quicker it breaks down. To feel fuller for longer, and to be kinder to your skin, the lower the number the better!

Try to eat low/medium GI foods:

- Whole grain sources of fibre will always be lower GI than their white counterparts (e.g. white/brown rice, white/brown bread Sweet potato is a great source of tonnes of nutrients and is low GI.
- Berries and most fruits are low GI. Berries are a great source of anti- oxidants too and they provide a lovely sweetness that you may be missing in a low GI diet.
- Dark chocolate with a high percentage of cocoa (full of antioxidants too).
- Non-starchy veg are low GI, e.g. peppers, salad veg (rocket and lettuce), mushrooms, baby corn (regular corn is a high-starch veg), broccoli, carrots (also a source of beta-carotene), cauliflower, cucumber (this is a high-water content food which is good for skin hydration), tomatoes, bean sprouts and beetroot – there are lots of them and you won't be stuck for choice.
- Legumes (e.g. beans, lentils and chickpeas) are a great low GI food as they usually provide us with bundles of protein and fibre too.
- Porridge is a low GI breakfast hero.

High GI foods to avoid:

- White bread, 'white' products of any kind
- Baked potatoes (according to Harvard University's *Harvard Health Publications*, a 150-gram baked potato has a GI of approximately 85 while a 150-gram boiled potato has a GI of approximately 50)
- Watermelon
- Dates
- Sugar snacks – be wary of cereals and cereal bars that appear healthy but are loaded with refined sugar
- Sweets
- Milk chocolate

Sugar Detox

To get your skin to a good starting point, I recommend a sugar detox.

SHOCK HORROR. I know, I'm saying the same!

By this, I mean trying to cut refined sugar from your diet entirely for a four-week period. This is presuming it's safe for you to do so – if you have any dietary concerns, check with your doctor. We suggest that it takes twenty-eight days for any new skincare regime to take effect and cutting out sugar will reduce a lot of the inflammation so your skin can start to heal.

Week 1 – try and go without added sugar.

Week 2 – go without processed sugar.

Week 3 – observe your mood, skin, healing, energy, etc. in your skin diary.

Week 4 – attempt zero sugar (yes, even fruit but only for a week).

In an ideal world, we'd cut refined and processed sugars forever, but do it for at least four weeks and measure the difference to your skin with your skin diary.

A lot of the damage caused by sugar, your AGEs for example, is cumulative because it goes on for a long time and so takes a while to undo. This is why an eye cream alone won't tackle all on the skin agenda. While sugar shouldn't really be in the body at all, I don't think it's entirely necessary – or even doable – to cut even naturally occurring sugars from your diet in the long term. I, for one, would be miserable. Instead, just monitor your sugar intake for this four-week period and be aware, going forward, of the effects that sugar can have on your skin. This is why we like being accountable for our diets in our skin diaries because when it's written down, there's no denying it.

Beyond the four weeks, don't deny yourself fruits as they are a great source of antioxidants. Just watch the refined foods. Lots of refined sugar in our diet means a cycle of inflammation that doesn't end. And if you're not getting anywhere with products but you're still consuming high volumes of sugar, you're probably wasting your money.

Dairy

Another topic that comes up a lot when we talk about food and the skin is the *D* word: dairy.

The relationship between dairy and the skin – acne in particular – has long been contested. Studies and research on this spans from the 1940s and 1950s. However, many of these studies were based on the subject's own assessment of their acne, which is not considered reliable. It remains a very difficult connection to prove but experts worldwide agree that regardless of why or how it happens, there does appear to be a correlation between dairy (specifically cow's milk) and the severity of acne. The most popular theory is that it has to do with the hormones found in cow's milk and how these hormones affect our skin. A

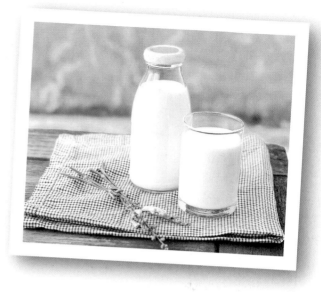

recent study has shown that skimmed milk has proven to be slightly worse when it comes to acne and it is thought to be due to lower oestrogen in the milk than in full-fat milk. I am not a nutritionist. I do, however, witness hundreds of results in clients of the Nerd Network that would suggest there is truth in this.

And despite clinical research having proved inconclusive, I have seen the effects of going dairy-free on people's skin. We've had clients who have tried everything – cosmetic skincare, cosmeceutical skincare, peels, antibiotics, hormonal medication and Roaccutane – but who only found relief when they made the switch to non-dairy alternatives.

Disclaimer: This might not work or be necessary for everyone, however, as I feel that skincare needs to be tackled from several angles. But high-dairy diets affect some of our clients and, when they limit their intake, their acne, congestion, eczema, etc. is massively reduced. These clients went from a persistent grade two or three (which is moderate to severe acne) down to a grade one or the odd spot. If you are at your wit's end with acne it's worthwhile trying to reduce your dairy intake, as long as you ensure you are getting your calcium from another source. The purpose of this action is trying to figure out the internal cause – technically, topical products will be able to minimise what the issue looks like on the outside and perhaps completely aid the issue if it is one that can be aided from the outside, but these products cannot stop your body from reacting to dairy, if dairy is an issue for you.

Going dairy-free should be done in conjunction with a skincare routine and if you're unsure if dairy affects you, please consult your doctor. This not dairy scaremongering. I am simply imparting what I have observed personally and professionally.

Alcohol and Caffeine

Sugar is not the only sure-fire enemy. There's also alcohol. All nights out cancelled … NOW!

Put simply, alcohol dehydrates your skin, just like caffeine. Alcohol is a diuretic and, as such, it sucks the moisture out of your skin. After a night out or an evening in with a few drinks, you might notice that your skin will be zapped of all its usual plumpness and freshness. You might also notice what we refer to as the 'Rudolph effect' in the bathroom mirror – alcohol consumption causes a release of histamine which causes flushing in the skin. Alcohol inflames the skin and the skin's tissue, leading to systemic inflammation (throughout the entire body rather than in one localised area) and thus encourages a skin reaction or flushing of the skin.

Because alcohol dehydrates the skin, it can lead to lines and wrinkles that will be visible almost immediately – we call these drink wrinkles 'drinkles'. Alcohol can also trigger inflammation and, in particular, irritates rosacea. It's commonly thought that alcohol is a cause of rosacea, but this is untrue. However, while enjoying a few cold ones doesn't leave you in imminent danger of developing rosacea, if you're already a sufferer of this condition, alcohol can exacerbate the symptoms.

Caffeine is also a diuretic so, like alcohol, it dehydrates us. Caffeine narrows blood vessels which can stop vital nutrients and oxygen from being delivered to the skin cells, which is why excessive caffeine drinkers have a greyish pallor. That said, when applied topically (as some skincare products contain caffeine), it can stimulate blood vessels from the outside to energise the skin and reduce the appearance of dark circles. Put it on, not in. I know you're telling me how lovely it tastes and how much you'd miss it! But try reducing your intake to one cup a day anyway.

Processed Foods

It is not so much that processed foods alone are actively bad for the skin, it's more that, generally speaking, they just aren't good and don't provide us with much nutritional value.

They increase inflammation as we know.

They tend to contain high amounts of salt, and salt is often a key culprit when it comes to puffy eyes because the salt causes our bodies to retain fluid which may result in some swelling. Too much salt can also lead to high blood pressure which can affect collagen production. (Isn't it all so positive?)

They're empty calories with little to no nutritional content.

They may be fast and convenient and suited to our lifestyle – but they're not adding any value to our health.

I find it interesting to observe how we look after babies – we give them only the best, so why not us as adults? When did plastic tube-shaped cheese become good for us?

Within processed foods, watch out for bad fats. Watch out for the word 'hydrogenated' on labels. Also known as trans fats, these are a by-product of a process called hydrogenation that is used to turn healthy oils into solids, to prevent them from going off. They are known to cause inflammation, unlike good fats such as polyunsaturated fats and monounsaturated fats. Within the realm of processed foods, you also have simple carbs, such as processed white breads that have had their vitamins and fibre rinsed from them, and salt-packed foods, which dehydrate us and thus our skin.

In an ideal world, you would avoid sugar as much as possible, and cut right down on alcohol and be mindful of our intake of processed foods (but hey, life gets in the way sometimes and we want to enjoy ourselves too).

If you are concerned about specific foods affecting your skin, I urge you to seek professional advice and go for intolerance testing. These tests are a great indicator of what may be causing more specific skin concerns or triggering certain conditions. Intolerance testing will take away a lot of the guess work for you. Then, when you're clear on any specific intolerances, you can come back to this guide as a general steer on skin-loving nutrition. It is a guide that can help you to understand your body's ability to react to food.

What foods are good for skin?

So, having addressed the baddies above, let's look at the nutrients found in certain foods that benefit the skin directly. These include Vitamin A, Vitamin C, essential fatty acids (EFAs) and antioxidants. Water is also key.

Vitamin A

'A' is the first letter of the alphabet and in my opinion the first vitamin to consider applying to your skin. It is one of the few vitamins that causes a physical change in the skin at a cellular level. Our skin can become deficient in its own Vitamin A due to UV exposure, even through the clouds, so we usually do not have enough of it to begin with. Our reservoir becomes depleted. Vitamin A is a necessary component for the function of all the cells within the skin. When we are deficient in Vitamin A, our *stratum corneum* becomes thickened and rougher and the living layer of the skin doesn't do as much because of sluggish cell division. The skin will feel rough and coarse and will be lacklustre in appearance. Pigmentation, or the overproduction of pigment, is more common in those deficient in Vitamin A, as is acne, because the skin is not proliferating properly (exfoliating at the rate at which it should, i.e. the 28-day cycle) and our skin also won't heal to its best ability.

Vitamin A is vital for all types of cells within our skin to function properly and enable it to carry out all its processes, such as healing, regeneration, exfoliating and its protective processes. Vitamin A will help to protect your skin from losing elasticity, from lax pores (pores that are loose and dilated), from hyperpigmentation and, to some extent, from acne.

For good sources of Vitamin A, many reach for carrots and sweet potatoes, which contain carotenoids in the form of beta-carotene which must be converted into Vitamin A in the body. Liver is a phenomenal source of Vitamin A, probably the best one, with turkey liver coming out on top (though liver for dinner isn't top of everyone's wish list). Orange-coloured vegetables also contain beta-carotene, but the amount of Vitamin A that ends up in the body because of conversion is low compared to that which you get from liver. Beta-carotene is an antioxidant in nature so boosting this is also providing you with protection from free radicals.

If you're pregnant, it is said that you should cut down on Vitamin A. Consult your doctor for more on this. If you're not currently pregnant, load up on:

- liver (direct Vitamin A)
- sweet potato (beta-carotene)
- pumpkin (beta-carotene)

- carrots (beta-carotene)
- squash (beta-carotene)
- kale (beta-carotene)
- goats cheese (direct Vitamin A)
- apricot (beta-carotene)
- eel (direct Vitamin A) Why not?!

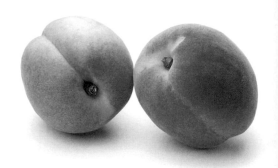

In general, the RDA of vitamin A for men is 0.7mg and for women is 0.6mg.

Vitamin E

We've long been told that Vitamin E is good for our skin (thank The Body Shop) and the reason it's been so popular is because of its hydrating and healing properties. Vitamin E is a fat-soluble nutrient that works as an anti-inflammatory agent within the skin and anything that can combat inflammation is always a good thing. It's also an antioxidant, so that's more armour against those free radicals (as well as being an all-round immunity booster).

You'll find Vitamin E in:
- wheatgerm and sunflower oil
- almonds
- hazelnuts
- sunflower seeds
- kale
- avocado
- sweet potatoes
- tomatoes

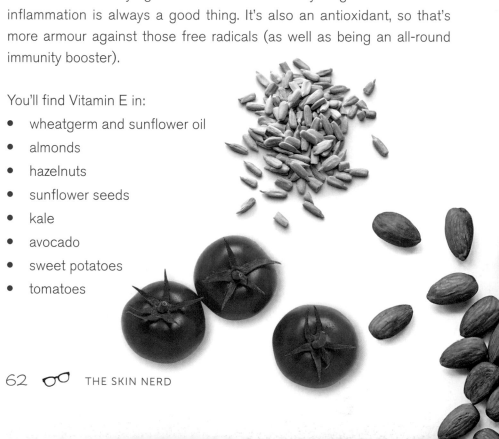

Vitamin D

Vitamin D is essential not just for the prevention of osteoporosis, but as more and more skin-specific research shows, it's necessary for beautiful-looking skin too. It is believed to increase elasticity and bounce, minimise acne (because of its anti-inflammatory properties), stimulate collagen production, lessen the appearance of lines and dark spots, and generally enhance radiance. Vitamin D is another powerful antioxidant and is said to be important for the control of the natural immune protective mechanisms of the skin. Vitamin D is something our body creates naturally when exposed to sunlight, but, over time, the body's ability to create Vitamin D lessens (in fact, it is said to go down 50 per cent from the age of twenty to seventy), which means you'll need extra Vitamin D as you get older.

When we age, our skin thins, which means that older skin finds it more difficult to create Vitamin D through (limited) exposure to sunlight. Bioactive Vitamin D (aka Vitamin D that can have an effect on living things) is essential for the formation of the skin's barrier. Vitamin D is also thought to have a positive effect when it comes to healing wounds.

The truth is you only need to have a coin-sized amount of skin exposed to sunlight for twenty minutes to get the adequate amount of Vitamin D, so don't fool yourself into thinking that you can bake yourself all day and bank it up. When you've hit those twenty minutes, your body stops making it – after that, you're just damaging your skin.

So get your twenty minutes in your twenties, but, as you get older, introduce more Vitamin D-rich foods as your body will need more of it.

Ingest Vitamin D via supplements as well as the following foods:

- tuna
- salmon
- eggs
- soya milk
- fortified orange juice

Vitamin C

Unlike Vitamin D, we don't make Vitamin C in our bodies at all, so we're fully reliant on food sources for our supply.

Vitamin C, as you now know, is a potent antioxidant. In fact, Vitamin C is a free radical scavenger and actively hunts them down. It also is a key component in the regulation of collagen being created in the skin so it can keep your skin looking plump and young for longer.

Vitamin C in our diets is also thought to fight against transepidermal water loss, successfully keeping our skin hydrated rather than losing moisture because of a compromised *stratum corneum* and superficial skin layer. It does this by locking the moisture levels into the skin in a sealant action and preventing our internal water reservoir from evaporating as rapidly.

Vitamin C also aids in the health of blood vessels and so may be a mode of prevention against broken capillaries by strengthening capillary walls. It also reduces redness in the skin.

Interestingly, there are plenty of foods that have more Vitamin C than oranges:

- red and green peppers
- kale
- strawberries

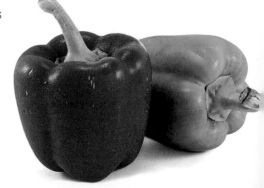

- kiwi
- citrus fruits
- tomatoes
- dark leafy greens
- cauliflower
- pineapple, which also contains bromelain, a digestive enzyme that will help in the breakdown of foods
- mango
- Brussels sprouts
- herbs, such as parsley, thyme and basil.

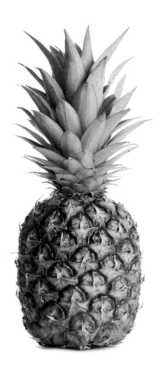

B vitamins

Why are Vitamin B or Vitamin B complex supplements marketed for those who are stressed? Well, basically, stress depletes your body's reservoirs of Vitamin B, possibly leaving you deficient. Vitamin B doesn't fix stress (if so, I'd be gobbling it up by the handful too), but it does help to replenish your stores of Vitamin B after stress has ravaged them.

In all, there are eight B vitamins, some of which have their own nicknames to make things extra confusing: Vitamin B1 (thiamin), Vitamin B2 (riboflavin), Vitamin B3 (niacin), Vitamin B5 (pantothenic acid), Vitamin B6 (has no nickname, wasn't popular in school), Vitamin B7 (biotin), Vitamin B9 (folic acid) and Vitamin B12.

Thiamin (Vitamin B1) is another vitamin we don't make as hooman beings, but it is crucial for the regeneration of collagen within the skin. It is found in whole grains, beef, pork, eggs and legumes.

Riboflavin (Vitamin B2) is key for the reparation of tissues within the body, so it is key for healing wounds. In a study carried out on rats, wound healing was slower in the rats that were deficient in riboflavin. It is found in: milk and dairy products, mushrooms, cooked spinach, Corn Flakes (yes, specifically Corn Flakes are very high in B2), liver, eggs and tempeh (a soy product).

Niacin (Vitamin B3, or niacinamide when it is in its most skin beneficial form) is a skingredient known for its lightening, brightening and hydrating qualities. It contributes to cellular energy in skin cells and can help to repair cell DNA. It also stops pigment from travelling in the skin. It is found in portobello mushrooms, potatoes, bran flakes/cereals, porridge, cottage cheese, liver, chicken, turkey, beef, lamb, pork, pumpkin, tempeh and peanuts.

Pantothenic acid (Vitamin B5) is thought to be helpful in reducing acne. The research on this isn't yet confirmed but a 2014 study in New York has shown that it may help, so it's something to keep in mind. Pantothenic acid is found in beef liver, shiitake mushrooms, sunflower seeds and chicken.

Vitamin B6 can help to regulate our hormones. If you're prone to hormonal acne, which appears just before or after your period or at specific points of your cycle (good time to check in on your skin diary), this vitamin could be beneficial. Good sources of Vitamin B6 include liver, chickpeas and Atlantic salmon (farmed or wild).

Biotin (Vitamin B7), is part of the structure of keratin, which is a key part of the skin. It is what makes the skin tough, resilient and not just soft goo that sits atop your other organs. Your nails and hair are also made up of keratin, which is why it is known for the strength of these too. It has been shown that biotin (via food and supplement form) is beneficial in the case of those who are deficient in it. However, there are few large-scale studies that have proven much when it comes to biotin supplementation in those who are not deficient. If you are not deficient in B7, you'll still want to make sure you're getting some of it through meat, egg yolks, salmon, beef liver, sweet potato, sunflower seeds, soy, wheat bran, avocado and spinach.

Vitamin B12 plays a role in the production of new cells. A deficiency of B12 can lead to pigmentation and markings on the nails. It also helps the body with how it uses protein too, and this means healthy skin cells. However, researchers in the University of California have published research in *Science Translational Medicine* showing that vitamin B12 can change the way skin reacts to acne bacteria in some people. This means that those who don't usually get acne could develop it.

It is important to not be deficient in Vitamin B12, as this deficiency plays a role in pigmentation, however, having it in excess may not be beneficial to the skin.

This is why it is important to be in tune with your body and keep diaries of symptoms and how you're feeling. If you think you have a Vitamin B12 deficiency, you should speak to your GP. Vitamin B12 is found in beef, lamb or veal liver, mussels and oysters.

Essential fatty acids

Essential fatty acids (EFAs) are referred to as 'essential' for a reason – your body needs them to function.

While your body already does a pretty good job of synthesising most of the fats it needs from your diet, there are two – linoleic acid and alpha-linoleic acid – that are not produced by the body naturally, so we need to get these via foods. These basic fats are used to build the specialised fats, omega 6 and omega 3 fatty acids, which are required by all the cells in your body in order to function normally.

Omega 6 (linoleic acid) is found in leafy vegetables, peanuts, grains, seeds, vegetable oils and meat. It's usually pretty easy to get enough omega 6 from your diet.

On the other hand, omega 3 (alpha-linoleic acid) is harder to get through the diet and you may need to be mindful of your intake. You'll find omega 3 in salmon, mackerel, mungo beans, edamame, linseeds, walnuts, hazelnuts, flaxseed and wheatgerm. You also

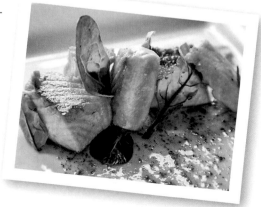

need to ensure that you're balancing your omega 6 and omega 3 in order to keep that homeostasis that we know is so important.

In terms of the skin, EFAs are responsible for the regulation of the cell membrane. They are vital for keeping water and nutrients within the skin cells while allowing bad things out. This minimises the appearance of ageing, dryness and cellulite too. Interestingly, these fats also help when excessive oiliness and congestion is an issue, because EFAs aid the proliferation process, cleansing the skin of fats and oils that would clog pores if not dealt with.

In general, EFAs balance our moisture levels. As you get older, your body struggles to retain moisture in its cells, so upping your EFA intake can help to counteract this. omega 3s help with signs of accelerated ageing in the skin and omega 6 is great for sensitivities, sensitisation and inflammatory skin disorders, such as eczema, psoriasis and rosacea.

Water and EFAs

The subject of water and skin has sometimes been controversial, with some skincare professionals suggesting that drinking water delivers no visible benefits to the skin.

This is only partly true.

The truth is, you won't see the benefits of drinking water in your skin unless you're eating your EFAs, which repair cell membrane to successfully hold the water into the skin, keeping it hydrated.

You can drink all the water you like but, unfortunately, it won't remain inside your skin unless you are also strengthening your skin's barrier and individual cells with EFAs.

I like to use a water balloon analogy to explain this. Imagine an empty water balloon. Your water balloon is your skin cell wall. If the wall is intact and you fill up the balloon with water, the water remains inside. The balloon won't burst. However, not eating enough EFAs is the same as the water balloon having a leak, so the water then leaks out.

If we are eating our EFAs, then water will help to keep the skin from becoming dry, tight and flaky. Dehydrated skin is less resilient and more prone to wrinkles, whereas hydrated skin looks plump. One study showed that drinking just half a litre of water per day increased blood flow to the skin which means more oxygen is reaching the skin, which we know is great for the skin (in the short term). It also boosted nutrients to each cell.

One to two litres is usually in and around the amount of water recommended by healthcare professionals. This is enough to keep our eyes and our joints nice and moist, to get rid of waste and toxins, and to hydrate skin cells.

Common signs of dehydration include a dry mouth, lips or sore eyes. (Your eyes need water to stop them from drying out. Have you ever been so dehydrated that you can HEAR yourself blink? That's not a good sign.) Other signs would be headaches with little other explanation, dark wee (you want a pale-yellow or clear wee, not sunflower yellow or anything darker), tiredness and dizziness.

Skin dehydration test

When it comes to skin hydration, my favourite test is the pinch test. All you have to do is pinch the back of your hands for a few seconds. If the skin bounces right back to where it was, you are hydrated. If it takes a second or two, that's a clear sign that your skin (and you) are dehydrated. Alternatively, feel your shin bones. If the skin there drags or pulls, it is dehydrated.

Beta-glucan

Beta-glucan is a lesser-known skin hero. It is a polysaccharide, which are chains of monosaccharides, which are small carbohydrates. Beta-glucan helps with the structure of cells and gives the body energy.

It is also renowned for its healing abilities, typically found in sensitive-skin topical ingredients. It's an antioxidant and helps to reduce unnecessary irritation and inflammation at a cellular level by helping the immune system to handle unwanted intrusions (such as stress or illness that can then affect the skin) better. It also minimises the damage done by toxins and stress.

Though it is not as widely celebrated as Vitamins A or C, it's an ingredient that I rate highly and look for when I can. Beta-glucan is derived from the cell walls of various foods, usually mushrooms or yeast.

You'll find beta-glucan in:

- mushrooms, including the shiitake, maitake, reishi and oyster varieties
- oats
- barley
- algae

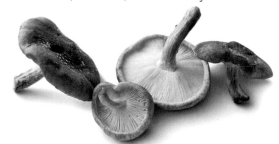

Antioxidants

As explained earlier, antioxidants are essential in the fight against oxidation and free radicals, countering, or at least delaying, the natural ageing process. As vitamin-like compounds found in plant-based food and extracts, antioxidants protect the collagen and other cells within the skin's architecture.

Vitamins C, E, D, beta-carotene and beta-glucan are all antioxidants in themselves, while other antioxidant-rich foods include goji berries, a known superfood and often the star of buddha bowls, smoothies and granola mixes, blueberries and cherries. Fruit and vegetables in general will usually provide you with antioxidant protection, so don't chuck out your oranges in lieu of only goji berries. In terms of how many antioxidants are enough, it's a case of the more the better. Send in an army of antioxidants as opposed to a lone soldier to fight the oxidative war.

Other antioxidant food heroes:

- tomatoes
- turmeric
- thyme
- ginger
- cranberries
- kidney beans
- dark chocolate – yes please!
- blueberries
- pecans

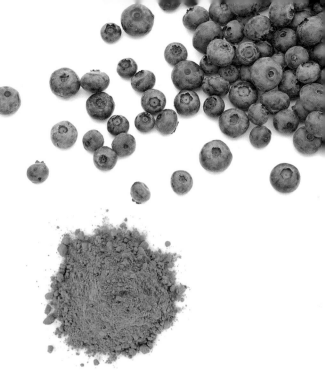

Zinc

While zinc may not be the first thing you think of when it comes to achieving beautiful skin, it's actually quite important as it enables more than 100 different enzymes in your body to function well.

Zinc is a trace mineral, which means that you only need small amounts of it each day (15mg is the average requirement, but pregnant and breastfeeding women will need a bit more – always check with your doctor to be sure to be sure). It's required for the function of all cell membranes and for new cell production.

Though not technically an antioxidant, zinc is a star player when it comes to your nutritional defence team for skin. It protects the fats in the skin (lipids), it reduces the formation of free radicals and it's also very important when it comes to healing. If you cut your skin, zinc rushes in to save the day, reducing inflammation and repairing the damage. It's also a known immunity booster and is said to reduce the amount of oil your skin produces naturally, meaning it could help in the fight against acne flare-ups. It is found in oysters, poultry and red meat, as well as beans, nuts and whole grains.

Phytonutrients

Phytonutrients refer to the beneficial chemical compounds found in plants. They occur naturally in certain foods but you'll also find them added to a lot of skincare products. Phytonutrients, unlike nutrients, are not essential to us as human beings but this doesn't mean that they aren't helping us in some way.

Carotenoids, such as beta carotene, are phytonutrients, as are flavonoids (which you'll find in tea, red wine – yay! – and apples) and resveratrol (found in peanuts, pistachios, red and white wine – again, yay!).

Lycopene and lutein are both phytonutrients too. Lycopene, found in tomatoes, can prevent the degradation of collagen in the skin and is also naturally photoprotective, meaning that it can help your skin with its defence against UV rays (but not enough to skip SPF!).

Lutein is a carotenoid that can protect the skin from the possible damage that blue light (HEV light, the type that is emitted by screens) may cause when applied topically. When ingested, it is fabulous for eye health too. You'll find it in dark leafy greens and egg yolks.

If you're wondering what the best phytonutrient you can get is, in my opinion, it's DIM (diindolylmethane), though it's not a word you'll hear a lot in skincare.

DIM is a phytonutrient found in cruciferous vegetables, such as Brussels sprouts, kale, broccoli and cabbage. It works to regulate oestrogen in the body and is often part of products known as 'oestrogen blockers' (the jury is out on whether or not it does truly block oestrogen). Not so much is known about DIM but, anecdotally, I've been a user and lover of that Advanced Nutrition Programme Accumax supplement, which includes DIM, for years and have personally seen results with it, as have many clients of mine who would have possibly had what is classed as hormonal acne. When you take it in supplement form, you get a super dose of greens, all of which contribute to beautiful skin. In food, try having a kale smoothie in the morning to get yours in.

One particular client of ours made a booking with Team Nerd for a consultation and must have cancelled two or three times because she was so upset about her skin and couldn't bear the thought of going makeup-free for her consult, even though it was important for us to see the skin without makeup. She started taking a DIM supplement and zinc as part of her new skincare routine, and within one month, I could hear the confidence come back to her voice when I phoned to check in. She'd already had a 10 per cent improvement – this is significant in an individual who suffered for years with a chronic condition. Eight to ten weeks later, her acne had gone down from a grade 3 to a grade 1, and she was well on her way to skin health. She was no longer red, swollen

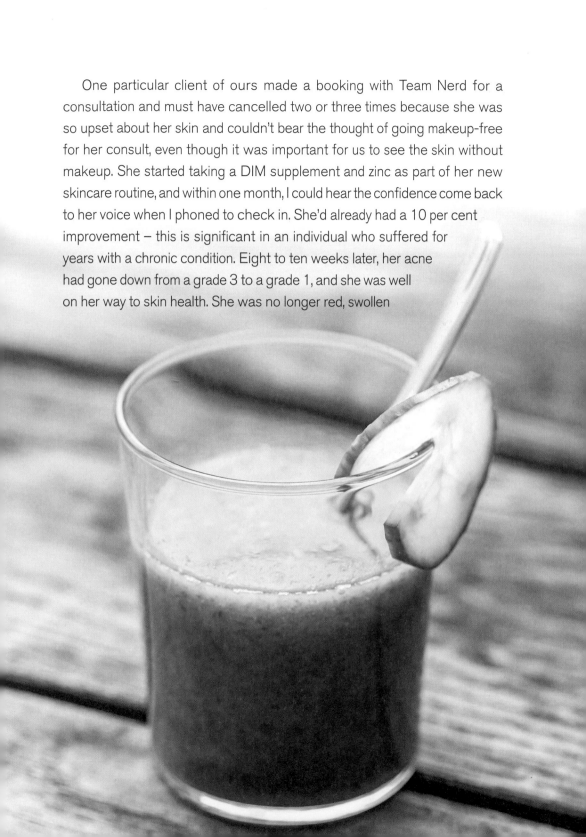

or tender, with angry-looking spots. Some spots were still appearing, but they were healing much faster. And if spots did come, they didn't leave a scar. Within ten weeks, she had a 50–60 per cent improvement. This timeframe is life-changing and realistic, particularly in a non-medical approach.

But, remember, this is not a one-time thing. When these super ingredients and phytonutrients start working for you, you can't just give them up. Incorporate them into your lifestyle for the long term.

Collagen

Collagen is one of the proteins that makes up the structure of the skin and other connective tissue in our bodies. It essentially makes up the dermis, the living layer of the skin below the epidermis. Collagen is what makes the skin firm and keeps it close to the contours of your face. Our own natural reservoir of collagen begins to deplete from the age of twenty-five. Fun and games, eh?

Collagen, when applied topically, is too large as a molecule to get anywhere near your dermis. However, it can be triggered via nutrients such as Vitamin A or Vitamin C or via clinical treatments. When ingested as hydrolysed collagen in supplements, it can have phenomenal results. When it is bio-available, it can be absorbed properly by the body. These are not for vegans or veggies though, as the sources of hydrolysed collagen are typically either marine or bovine.

Collagen supplements don't just include collagen. They often include high amounts of Vitamin C, which is essential for the skin's own production of collagen, alongside other ingredients that feed the skin from within. It's an ideal supplement for those with mature or ageing skin but can be used by everyone (but do check with your doctor).

The best collagen supplements, in my opinion, include IMAGE Skincare YANA Collagen Shots, Skinade and ZENii ProCollagen Supplements. I always look forward to learning about more!

The ideal skin diet

The goal is to give your skin as much variety of nutrients as you can because, essentially, every nutrient has at least one benefit to the skin whether directly or indirectly.

Now, before we go any further, let me remind you again that I am in no way shape or form a dietician or nutritionist. Before you make any drastic dietary changes (such as cutting out dairy for example), you should talk to your doctor, especially if you are on medication. What follows is my general nutritional recommendations for a good skin health day.

Start your day with something like mashed avocado on seeded bread – very millennial indeed – to get in your essential fatty acids, fibre and lots of other nutrients. Fibre is good for you in general but it specifically helps the skin by helping the gut. Remember the gut-skin axis/connection? We need fibre for good digestion. If we have bad digestion, our skin may suffer. Supplement your avo on toast with strawberries or an orange for Vitamin C, or some blueberries for their antioxidant benefits.

Another breakfast option that is good for the skin is unsweetened live yoghurt with strawberries and sprinkled with flaxseed. The live yoghurt is a probiotic (gut health!), the strawberries are high in Vitamin C and the flaxseed is great for EFAs.

I personally like a kale and quinoa burger (Strong Roots do an amazing one – delish!) for breakfast (yes, I'm odd) for all those B vitamins, Vitamin A, Vitamin C, fibre and protein.

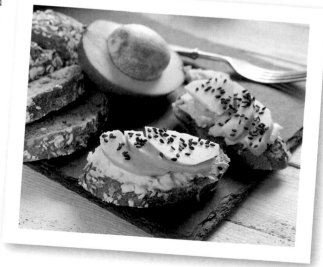

Carrots and hummus make a great healthy snack. Carrots are of course a great source of beta-carotene and though I like hummus more so for its taste – one of its main ingredients is chickpeas, which are high in protein and fibre too.

Protein is a major building block of the skin and is so important for healing and repairing damage. A palmful of almonds is a great high-protein snack, as are roast chickpeas and edamame beans and I always feel quite cultured eating this (just throw them in a hot oven – 180-200 degrees –for thirty or forty minutes and they get crispy).

Protein as a snack is great as it helps us to feel full, leaving less room for heavily processed snacks. If you've packed a protein-rich snack, you'll be less likely to take those cautious steps towards the vending machine.

Another snack option is apple and natural peanut butter (peanut butter that is not processed – the 'no added sugar, no-peanut-taste' kind of peanut butter). This will satisfy sweet cravings and is high in protein and fibre and contains Vitamin C too, and EFA omega-6 in the peanut butter. For other sweet kicks, fruit is naturally sweet and berries, like raspberries, strawberries and blueberries, are low GI but taste as sweet as anything. I mean, they ain't no Dairy Milk but I'd like lovely skin, please. Have a handful of berries and unsalted nuts like unsalted walnuts and cashews for an antioxidant boost. The nuts will help you feel full so you'll be less inclined to keep reaching for snacks in the first place.

For dinner, have salmon (oven bake it or steam it to retain the nutrients as much as possible) with sweet potato wedges for your beta-carotene, add some turmeric in your seasoning for its fab anti-inflammatory benefits but only a bit as it can be quite bitter. Turmeric is great with cayenne and a bit of salt and pepper. Pair it with kale, spinach and beetroot. Kale is high in Vitamin C and beta-carotene as well as being loaded with B vitamins. Spinach has beta-carotene and Vitamin C, and beetroot has Vitamin A and Vitamin C among others. Beetroot wedges = deliciousness on a plate.

My Mini Nerd (AKA Matt, my son) and I have a chart similar to a skin diary on our wall where we report to ourselves how many EFA-rich foods we've eaten, how much water we've drunk during the day and other things like that. The only person who can truly make sure if you're eating well is yourself – or your mum, in Matt's case. Seeing what you are eating visualised will help you understand what you need more or of or less of.

	Essential Fatty Acids	Protein	Good Carbs	Good Fats	Antioxidants	H20	Processed Foods
Mon							
Tues							
Wed							
Thurs							
Fri							
Sat							
Sun							

*We do agree with treats on Sunday, perhaps without going too bananas. Sunday is Skinday too so give it a treat externally with a masque or a facial massage.

Skin Diary Check-in:

Now you know the nutrients necessary for healthy skin, note in your skin diary what might be lacking as well as what you're getting plenty of. Is your protein intake what it should be? Could you introduce more Vitamin A-rich foods? →

Once you identify what you need more of, make a list of some foods that will help increase your intake and try to think of fun ways to introduce them into your diet. Maybe you'll come across a new recipe, or start drinking smoothies in the morning?

And think about your diet with your skin in mind – are there any obvious changes you could try to help with skin conditions you're experiencing?

Take a look at what you might need to cut back on – I know, it's hard. But maybe those three cups of coffee a day should become two … and then one. And it's probably time to stop adding those spoonfuls of sugar…

If you decide to take on the sugar detox challenge, note the results week by week.

Don't forget to take photos of your skin every two weeks so you can objectively track improvements. Save these images in a secret skin folder so nobody but you can take a peek.

Is a balanced diet enough?

At the Skin Nerd HQ, we don't claim to be nutritionists, but knowing what we know, we are huge advocates of a balanced diet (although what is balanced to one is not to another), complete with a wide range of skin-loving nutrients. We follow the dinner plate rule, which means you need carbs, protein, good fats and vegetables in the correct proportions on a daily basis. (We also follow this rule in skincare as there are core skingredients needed in traditional skincare, i.e. cleansers, serums and sunscreen.) This generally means 40–50 per cent vegetables, 20–25 per cent lean protein and 20–25 per cent starchy carbohydrates on your dinner plate. However, you may need more carbs if you carry out physical labour or more protein if you are on a particular fitness regime (consult a nutritionist if unsure).

Typically, the number of nutrients required (when you look at recommended daily allowances, etc.) is tailored towards the minimum needed for general health – the minimum. However, you need to have much more Vitamin C than what you can get in a recommended diet (which, some say, is the amount you need not to get scurvy) for it to have a true effect on your skin. For vitality and glowing skin, you need to up the ante across the RDA you'll find on labels. The RDA is the level you need in order to live without disease. We should be aiming for the ODA, or optimum daily allowance.

Supplements

One question I'm often asked is this: 'Is a balanced diet enough?' In my experience, not quite, though I wish it was. Your skin will benefit from the combination of a colourful, veg-rich diet and supplements. Rainbow plates result in healthy, bouncy, fresh-looking skin.

Supplements cannot be used in the place of food in your pursuit of skin health, but they can help. The reason I believe in the addition of supplements is because we live such fast-paced lives and experience such high amounts of stress, it's hard to know the levels of nutrition we're truly getting from your food. We overcook our food, we microwave it, we fry it, we horse it in without chewing thoroughly (affecting the way the nutrients are absorbed) and all of these things can deplete the value of the food.

Then, there's the challenge of getting higher volumes of nutrients into your diet: the fact that we're not always that hungry. What's more, the food you eat is only as good as the soil it's grown in. Without going too deep into agriculture, crop rotation is an issue. In the past, there would always be one dormant field which enabled the soil to rest, but, today, mainly because of demand, farmers can't rest their soil, so it's not as jam-packed full of minerals as it once was. C'est la vie.

Finally, you're only as healthy as the food that you can digest. It would be great if we could all eat food we had grown in our gardens as it would be pesticide- and herbicide-free. Unfortunately, this isn't possible and these things impact on the way your body will absorb the nutrients in your food.

So supplements, including probiotics for the gut, are a helping hand, delivering higher levels of nutrients than we'd get from food alone. They are *not* an alternative but should be taken in addition to a healthy diet. Just like with the Sunday papers, the weekly supplement is a bonus.

Even if we achieve a very balanced diet, it can be difficult for us to take in every single nutrient our body needs through food alone. Supplements give us the opportunity to top up our bodies and feed our skin with extra goodness.

Supplements require patience as it takes a while for the results to be seen, unlike the more immediate effects of, for example, a mask. It's different for everyone, but I would say it can take at least a month for supplements to take effect. Skin Accumax by Advanced Nutrition Programme (my go-to, as mentioned earlier) advise ninety days – but it could be three weeks; it could be twelve weeks. It depends on your levels of the nutrients in the first place, how much you already have in your diet and how your body metabolises them.

As the ingestible skincare market has exploded, there are now

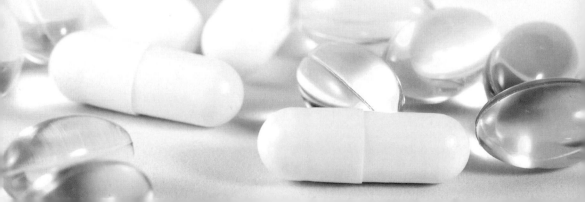

countless brands to choose from but here we will cover what you're looking for. In my work, I make sure I see before and afters ahead of recommending a brand to a client. I only offer brands from within the skincare sector, meaning the supplements are created purely for the skin, and will have an effect on the skin. It's important when we are looking for skin health that these supplements are tested for skin results and not just for general overall health results. I do understand that body health is vital but my goals are skin goals!

Whatever brand you go with, you need to know that there are two kinds of supplements: water-soluble for those who hate swallowing tablets, and capsule form – which you use is really just a personal choice. My rule of thumb is to look for case studies, testimonials and those before and after pics; more often than not, these are a better guide than reading about clinical trials.

You should always be mindful of taking supplements with or directly after food, otherwise you might experience what I call the omega burps, the sexiest aftertaste and belch known to man. (I suggest keeping these for a first date. Now that is an endurance and a half!) Though good skincare supplements will have many benefits, they can cause indigestion and a heartburn-like sensation if you don't take them near meal times. Take yours in between meals and you might suffer a fate like one member of Team Nerd. She took a powdery supplement a little bit too late after a meal whilst on a date. The capsule burst in her throat and her mouth filled with powder. Her date was asking her what was wrong and she couldn't respond because if she did she would have puffed a mouthful of white powder at his face. She explained after but he looked at her funny for

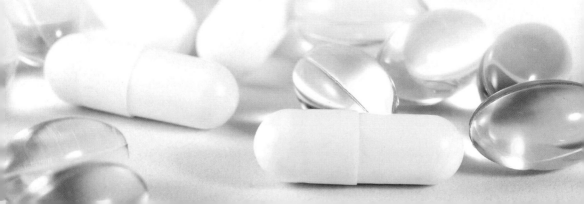

the rest of the evening. Don't worry, they are still together so it is not the end of the world – but it's not ideal either. Every brand has different and specific methods and times to take the supplement so always follow the relevant instructions.

When looking for supplement ingredients, consider additional EFAs. Once a week is simply not enough fish to get your EFAs in (especially omega 3) and fish fingers or a battered chip shop cod do *not* count. Then, you want to add more antioxidants, Vitamin A, Vitamin C, probiotics (which boost immunity and promote gut health which improves our healing ability) and digestive enzymes (which help to break down our food more easily).

Is there one wonder supplement for all of the above? Usually, you won't get all of these in one tablet but ZENii ProClear gets pretty close. However, if you're taking an all-in-one, it's important to consider how much (in terms of dosage) the manufacturer was able to get into one capsule. You're going to get higher amounts of one thing if it is in a supplement pretty much on its own.

Maybe, however, you'll be like me, and need six different supplements per day – it all depends on what you're trying to do. I take:

- **Omegas** (Udo's Choice or Advanced Skin Nutrition omegas), to control oil and hydrate my skin from the inside out. I take two with dinner.
- **Vitamin A** (Advanced Skin Nutrition Accumax), to prevent future spots and balance my hormones. I take one to two a day with dinner.
- **Vitamin C** (Biocare Vitamin C 1000), 1000mg Vitamin C daily, again one tablet with dinner. I take this as a powerful antioxidant and immune system booster.
- **Diindolylmethane (DIM)** (Advanced Nutrition Programme Skin Accumax) for regulating hormones as above and assisting the inner rocky fluctuations that trigger hormone-related skin issues.

- **Probiotics** (I alternate between Udo's Choice, Symprove and ZENii), for optimal gut health.
- **Digestive enzymes** (Advanced Skin Nutrition Digestive Enzyme), one before each meal to make sure I'm digesting my food properly and absorbing all of my nutrients.

Generally speaking, I adore the Advanced Nutrition Programme, with whom I worked as a trainer, as well as Biocare, Solgar, Symprove Probiotics, Udo's Choice, ZENii, Cell Nutrition.

It's OK to take more than one supplement at once, but make sure you're not getting toxic levels of anything – be especially careful with Vitamin A. You shouldn't be getting more than 300,000 IU (international units) of Vitamin A per day as this can lead to Vitamin A toxicity. Also, you shouldn't take Vitamin A supplements if you are pregnant or breastfeeding. Post-baby and breastfeeding, take all the A you can get because babies age you. Teens … no comment!

Taking multiple supplements just means multiple benefits and targeting concerns from all angles. Ain't nothing wrong with that.

- If ageing is your concern, go for Vitamin A, omegas, Vitamin C and collagen supplements.
- If acne/oily skin is your worry, go for Vitamin A, DIM, zinc, omegas and probiotics.
- For pigmentation help, choose Vitamin A and Vitamin C.
- For dry skin, flaky skin and inflammatory skin conditions, you'll want omegas, Vitamin A, Vitamin C (for redness) and Accumax or Pro Clear from ZENii.

Whatever your concern, the following taken as supplements are beneficial for everyone: probiotics, digestive enzymes, omegas, Vitamin A, Vitamin C, collagen and antioxidant supplements. These are the core nutrients everyone could benefit from and taking them won't cause any harm. Beyond the specific ingredients, look for a supplement with a high rate of bioavailability (the rate at which the nutrients will be absorbed by your body). If a supplement has a high rate of bioavailability/absorption and a fab mode of doing it, the producer will probably a) rave about it on the packaging and marketing and b) have lots of info on it on their website. Research the brand as much as possible – heck, you can even email their customer service team asking questions! Two things to look for are whether a brand's supplements are lab-tested and tested on humans.

The thing is, it's not just the food you eat that your skin depends on, but your body's ability to digest it, absorb and distribute it. The better the quality of the food or the supplement, the easier it will be on your gut and the more you (and your skin) will benefit from it. Does it fizz? If so, walk away, nerd. Walk away.

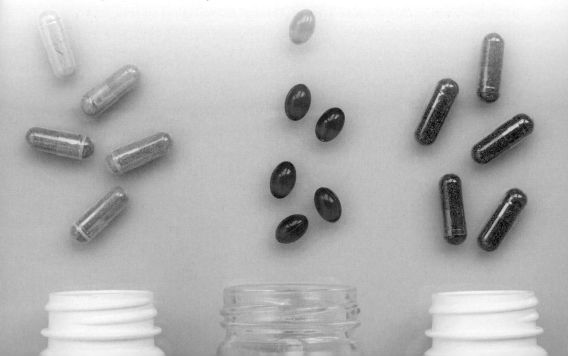

Find out as much as you can about the manufacturer, about where they source their ingredients, whether or not they use anti-caking agents (that stop the ingredients from binding together) that you'd prefer not to be ingesting and find out about their quality checks. Like anything in life, you want your supplements to be high quality. Check the levels of the ingredients and whether or not the ingredient list contains anything where it isn't clear what it is or what its purpose is. Take to Google with the specific anti-caking ingredients. Read the brand's website or speak to a representative. It is more of a hassle than just grabbing supplements off of a supermarket shelf but it is worth it. Is this a lot to expect from a non-expert? Yes, but it is how to ensure that you're using high-quality supplements! If you drink fizzy drinks, wine and dine, yet question putting supplements into your body, I'd rethink the overall picture.

What do I recommend?

From my own experience and from training hundreds of therapists and seeing their clients and our clients benefit, my favourite brands are (at the time of writing this book) Advanced Nutrition Programme and Yana from IMAGE Skincare. Both of these supplement brands are clinically proven and I have seen the results time and time again (not just others or with my clients but with myself). What you're getting here with either Advanced Nutrition Programme – whose hero product is Accumax – and Yana from IMAGE is high-potency ingredients with which you'll see a massive difference. In fact, a mahoosive one (which is Nerdie speak) – try it! It is only applicable for certain skin conditions though so stay educated.

Yana by IMAGE

Yana Daily Collagen Shots by IMAGE contain hydrolysed collagen peptides – which is collagen that has been treated so that it can be extracted and absorbed by the body, as the molecules are smaller in size. It reduces the appearance of wrinkles, increase the skin's elasticity and slows down how quickly we naturally lose our collagen. It contains Vitamin C to boost our skin's own production of collagen, biotin to help with skin strength, Vitamin B6 to tackle the breaking down of collagen within the skin as well as an antioxidant complex that contains HA (hyaluronic acid, also a laugh a minute), green tea leaf extract, acai fruit extract and pomegranate fruit extract.

Yana is taken as a shot (shots, shots, shots, but not the type most people think of!) once a day. I advise my clients to drink this shot in the morning with breakfast. You can expect smooth, firm, hydrated, younger-looking skin within just a month of starting to take it. It is truly fab for skin ageing (which as you now know, begins at twenty-five). Drink it cold and it is as tasty as can be.

Skin Accumax by Advanced Nutrition Programme

Skin Accumax are incredible supplements designed to create hormonal homeostasis which is great for acne sufferers. They are packed with Vitamins A, C and E but the magic ingredient is DIM (Diindolylmethane) which, by now, you'll know as one of my all-time favourite skingredients. The thing is, to get high levels of DIM into your diet, you'd need to be eating your broccoli by the truckload.

With Skin Accumax, you can expect a reduction of size and redness of spots, as well as them clearing in general – though it does depend on your skin in the first place. At the very least, it will help to bring spots from a level where they are red, inflamed, painful and very infected to being smaller, less painful, less red and just less vicious. With Skin Accumax, they recommend that you take two capsules twice a day (morning and evening, after eating) for a minimum of fourteen weeks until you see a significant difference in your skin and then you should drop to one capsule twice a day.

Probiotic supplements

As hoomans, we are covered and filled with bacteria – but not all bacteria is bad. Like the word 'fat', it has become a word – and ingredient – thought of negatively, which should not be the case. Both our gut and our skin have incredibly complex ecosystems made up of many different types of microorganisms that essentially make sure that everything is working as it should.

When there is an imbalance of bacteria in the gut, it causes inflammation and this, in turn, can cause inflammation of the skin. In the words of the great Diana Ross, you're in the middle of a chain reaction. This connection between gut flora, which are the microorganisms that live in our gut, and the skin is known as the gut–skin axis. For example, studies have shown that those with rosacea are more likely to have a bacterial overgrowth of the small intestine and those who have inflammatory gut conditions are generally more likely to also have an inflammatory skin condition along with it.

Your balance of gut bacteria is altered through daily life. Medication (specifically antibiotics) that is taken regularly can upset the delicate ecosystem of your gut, as can stress and not sleeping properly. By taking probiotic supplements, you can help to repair the balance of bacteria in your gut, and thus stop the gut inflammation from occurring in the first place. This is why taking probiotic supplements is so important, especially for those with rosacea, eczema and even severe congestion – all hoomans in fact.

I have seen people try everything when it comes to topical skincare and see little effect, then when we introduce a probiotic supplement once or twice a day, they see a phenomenal difference. We refrain from saying 'I told you so' unless it is a family member, but we are still thrilled that they are en route to results.

In terms of brands and options on the market right now, I adore Symprove as it is live bacteria in a drinkable form. Symprove isn't freeze dried and reactivated as many probiotic-based supplements are. Its delivery system means that the digestive system doesn't see the live and active bacteria in the formulation as food and so doesn't attack it. This means it can pass straight through the stomach to start work colonising your gut bacteria. It also contains four different probiotic strains. It's not the easiest to manage as it needs to be stored in a fridge and it is not the most appealing to the eye. My tip is to close your eyes and drink it. Daily. It is also expensive but if you would buy a Zara top and wear it once, don't tell me that a tonic at €3 a day is expensive. Your body is your home. I truly see differences in my immunity, my skin's healing ability and my own energy levels when I'm taking this against when I'm not (ideally I should be taking this all of the time, but being a hooman myself, sometimes I fall off the supplements wagon!). It also improves my digestion. It's expensive but it's really brilliant. Udo's Choice is another option, and Optibac is a more affordable probiotic option. Affordability is key. I also believe in prioritising differently, depending on your key concerns.

Topical probiotics

What you might not realise is that you can also take probiotics topically. Your skin also has its own microbiome that is separate to that of your gut. Given that your skin is not protected by fat, tissue and skin, which the gut is cocooned within, it is a lot easier for its natural bacterial balance to be harmed.

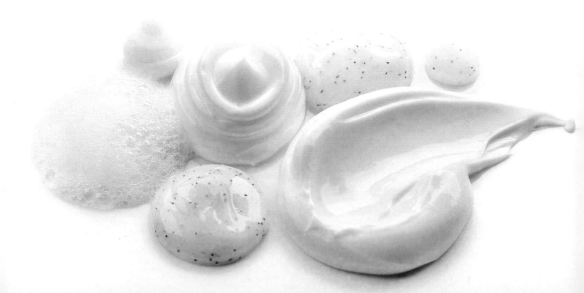

Good bacteria are what make up the skin's acid mantle – its protective Tupperware lid layer – that stops harmful bacteria and viruses from attacking the skin. It is a diversity of skin bacteria that is thought to battle eczema, rosacea and acne, so topical probiotics are like fertiliser for the beneficial bacteria that may help to stave off breakouts and flare-ups of these conditions.

But probiotics aren't only beneficial to those with 'problem' skin. Topical probiotic skincare can reduce the appearance of fine lines and wrinkles and speed up your skin's processes of reparation. Recall that ageing slows down the body's rate of repair.

I'm sure your mind has wandered to the four-pack of Activia in your fridge, but there is no point applying probiotic yoghurt like a mask as the molecules of yoghurt are simply not small enough to penetrate the skin – and you will just smell funny when it warms up. If your skin and your body is OK with dairy, introducing probiotic yoghurts into your diet won't hurt, but they can be packed full of sugar so look out for this. There are alternatives for skin probiotics that work in conjunction with your skin's natural bacteria, unlike the ingestibles which are designed for bacteria in your gut. Both are bacteria, both designed for different locations.

You can colonise your skin's bacteria from the outside with probiotic skincare like Gallinée or Biofresh. These products contain topical probiotic ingredients that you can apply in cleansers, creams and masks. This would be either alternating with active skincare or as your main product (cleanser, mask or otherwise) and they could be used every day. Probiotic skincare is usually very helpful to those with sensitised skin as extrinsic factors have destroyed their skin's bacterial balance.

When will you see results? Supplements are slow burners. Advanced Nutrition Programme say that you sometimes need to take Skin Accumax for over three months to see a result but some see it in a few weeks. Consistency is key.

Skin Diary Check-in:

Are you taking any supplements?

What are they and what purpose do they serve? Are they high-quality? Have you noticed a difference since you started taking them?

If you add in a supplement such as Skin Accumax or omegas, note each day that you've taken them.

Track the changes with photos on a weekly basis.

Skin Types

Skin Types

Dry? Oily? Normal? Combination? We're all familiar with these categories but such generalised skin types are not my thing. In my nerdie opinion, they aren't comprehensive enough to point you in the right direction towards healthy skin. I'd rather treat and discuss skin concerns. The distinction between the two will become clearer soon.

Before we work on figuring out what your skin situation is, let's take a look at the different skin types.

The four pillar skin types date back to 1902 when cosmetics giant Helena Rubinstein first divided the skin into these categories. While it was revolutionary for its time, today I feel we can apply a far more accurate scientific criteria to the skin. That said, as these types are commonly referred to in the skindustry, I'll expand on these terms and then we can dive a little deeper.

Normal skin

With normal skin, your sebaceous glands secrete oil at a normal rate. Pore size is normal and small (the size of a pinprick), moisture content is good, texture is even and elasticity is good. You won't be aware of any oiliness or dryness. You won't have a sheen, but you may appear dewy from healthy skin, which is a good thing.

Dry skin

Generally speaking, if you struggle with dry skin you may have underactive sebaceous glands. You're not producing enough oil and therefore your skin appears dull and matte. The skin is fine and delicate. Moisture content with dry skin is poor, while the skin lacks suppleness and bounce.

Oily skin

The skin has many oil glands which secrete wax esters, triglycerides and squalene. These fats form a film to keep the moisture on the skin. Increased sebum results in oily skin and can be triggered by diet, stress and hormones. Genetics, again, may play a role. With oily skin you have typically overactive sebaceous glands, with shiny, thickened, coarse, enlarged pores. You'll struggle with a sluggish pallor and regular blackheads and spots may be present more often. For those with oily skin, oiliness can occur all over the body.

Combination skin

Combination skin is a mixture of either oily and normal skin, or dry and normal skin. It is unlikely that anyone would have a mixture of dry and oily skin; if you think you do, it may be oily mixed with dehydrated skin (I'll explain the difference between these shortly). If oily, you'd have it usually on the T-Zone (as we have more oil glands here) or in localised areas. Pore size may vary on different parts of the face.

Your Skin Barrier

Typically how oily or dry our skin is, even how sensitive it is, is determined by your skin's barrier and its condition. If you have normal skin, it means that the health of your skin barrier is good.

The skin barrier is at the root of most skin conditions. It is like a brick wall, with each brick held in place by a lipid (nerdie term for fat), and it keeps the good in and bad out. But the barrier can be weakened or damaged by harsh weather, detergents, acetone, chloride, prolonged water immersion (those of you who spend too long in a hot shower) and chemicals. Genetics can also play a part.

An impaired barrier can cause the skin to lose moisture or allow irritants to slip through, which can make the skin dry or sensitised. And though lathering the skin in thick creams may seem like its helping, it unfortunately doesn't do the work needed to resolve the issue. What does help is reducing exfoliation, wearing SPF and generally making efforts to shield your skin.

Beyond standard skin types

To understand how your own skin is performing and more importantly what it needs, I believe we need to go beyond the simplicity of oiliness versus dryness and also look at factors such as dryness versus dehydration, sensitisation or sensitivity versus resilience, pigment versus non-pigment, and accelerated collagen degradation versus collagen degradation. Worry not, I'll walk you through them.

My goal as The Skin Nerd is not to lean on the famous four but to analyse the skin further, so that we can arrive at the best possible conclusions.

Dryness versus dehydration

Dry skin is a skin type. Dehydrated skin is a skin condition that happens when your skin is lacking moisture. Dry skin lacks oils; dehydrated skin lacks water.

Dry skin is genetic. It is something you are born with and your skin will have always been dry, whereas dehydrated skin occurs as a result of lifestyle choices and, sometimes, neglect. Dehydrated skin can also be the fault of an impaired barrier, which leads to the skin losing moisture. If your skin is dehydrated, your lines will look more prominent, you'll look duller and your skin may feel tight, itchy and a bit irritated.

I often do a dehydration test in the mirror. If you scrunch up your nose and see little taut lines, this is usually a sign of dehydration. If you press on your cheek and push it upwards and see horizontal lines, this is another way of telling whether or not your skin is dehydrated. Dehydration is an issue for an awful lot of people as they don't get enough water and EFAs to keep the moisture levels in check. (See pinch test, p. 69)

Sensitisation or sensitivity versus resilience

Sensitive skin, like dryness, is genetic – something you're born with. Simply put, your skin is cautious and is more susceptible to reactions.

People often think that sensitive skin is a skin type, but it's actually more like a skin condition. Sensitive skin is dealing with chronic irritation and a heightened awareness of the skin's state. Ingredients and any new stimuli may trigger it. Sensitisation, on the other hand, is caused by lifestyle factors, be it overuse of products or neglecting the skin as an organ. Inflammation is the common denominator with sensitised or sensitive skin; those with this kind of skin are prone to spots, redness, rosacea and itchy skin.

Coming in from the cold to a severely heated home can sensitise the skin; not using SPF or moisturising can sensitise the skin; baby wipes and micellar waters can sensitise the skin; over-exfoliation, misuse of harsh skincare ingredients and super-hot showers can sensitise the skin. Drinking alcohol also sensitises the skin as it can dehydrate it.

It's easy enough to tell the difference between sensitive and sensitised skin. If your skin suddenly starts rejecting certain ingredients after years of accepting them willingly, it may have become sensitised. If your skin is sensitised, it may look thin, feel tight after cleansing and may be red, scaly or bumpy.

On the other end of the spectrum, when we speak of skin resilience, or someone who has resilient skin, we mean someone whose skin doesn't react easily or negatively. A resilient skin has a solid shield, with its barrier intact. The ironic aspect is that this skin will find it harder to get results with active ingredients because the barrier is doing preventing penetration!

Pigment versus non-pigment

Another thing I look for, beyond 'dry' or 'oily' or 'normal', is pigment versus non-pigment. We all have pigment in our skin to shield us from over-exposure to light, but when we expose ourselves to light for a prolonged period, we cause an enzyme activity that attempts to create an umbrella shield for the skin.

Pigment, or hyperpigmentation, is a darkening of the skin, tan or freckles. Non-pigment is a loss of pigment and, therefore, a loss of protection. Melasma is pigment mask (known as chloasma in pregnant women) where pigment appears in a butterfly fashion across the cheeks. Ephelides are freckles, as in genetic freckles that you have your whole life that fade after sun exposure, the ones that appear in the fair-skinned; age spots/sun spots/liver spots are all just colloquial terms for lentigos. None of these are caused by age or your liver, they are all sun-related damage. Older people have them because they have been alive longer and so have had more sun exposure!

Though it's something we've been conditioned to associate with beauty, a tan, which is pigmentation caused by sun exposure, is nothing more than a scar. The skin changes colour to defend itself. Melanin is key in shielding our skin. It is the barrier defence against light and is triggered by the skin which damages the DNA of the 'mother cell' (i.e. the cell found in the fifth layer of the epidermis where all skin cells are created), and alters the core so the skin cells made thereafter are pigmented. Pigmentation can also be caused by hormonal-related situations, such as puberty, taking the contraceptive pill, HRT, thyroid medication and pregnancy.

There are different kinds of pigmentation.

Melasma is one characterised by light, brown and grey patches of skin in sun-exposed areas often in the shape of a butterfly across the nose and cheeks.

Ephelides is the nerdie term for freckles. I love freckles, if they are indeed freckles; typically they are sun damage specks that we convince ourselves are freckles. Find a picture of yourself as a youngster, did you have them blowing out the candles of your third birthday cake? If not, it's sun damage. Ephelides are true freckles – solar lentigos or lentigines are the type caused by sun damage. Freckles are genetic and occur in those who do not have a lot of melanin in their skin in the first place, meaning they are not well-protected genetically from the sun. The freckles operate a bit like a warning sign to be careful of sun damage. If you always get

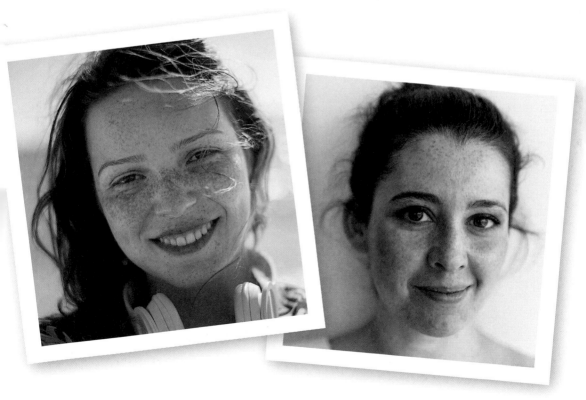

freckles, it's nothing to worry about usually but maybe up your SPF if they come about all of a sudden with no warning.

The majority of our clients will confuse their freckles with solar lentigos or sun damage.

If you were icy pale in your youth but now you're darker, your freckles are more likely to be lentigos. Hold up your inner arm to your face – this skin has not been as exposed unless you sunbathe constantly with your arms behind your head – I believe that this skin is a good guide in terms of the texture, clarity, and colour of our skin, were we protected from the elements.

We're largely obsessed with wrinkles, lines and pores yet, in my opinion, an even skin colour is the strongest indicator of a youthful appearance.

Non-pigment, or hypopigmentation, is exactly what it sounds like – a lack of pigment. It happens when melanocytes and melanin decrease in the skin or when we have less tyrosine, an amino acid that is used to make pigment. It will show up as patches or spots that are paler than the rest of us and is common in darker skin tones. Vitiligo is a commonly known form of hypopigmentation, famously afflicting the model Winnie Harlow, that occurs when melanocyte cells die.

Injury and trauma to the skin of any form can caused hypopigmentation, including sun damage, cuts, grazes, spots and chickenpox. It's not uncommon for it to occur because of poorly performed skin treatments, such as light-based therapy (like IPL, which can also cause hyper-pigmentation) or chemical peels.

IPL and Fraxel Laser are clinic-based hypopigmentation treatments but topical corticosteroids can also help. Alternatively, it can be treated in the inverse by lightening or bleaching the surrounding skin with lightening agents to help the hypopigmentation blend in with the skin around it.

For every pigment-related concern, use factor 50, broad spectrum sunscreen every day. It may help with the prevention of hypopigmentation and will help to stop it from getting worse. The global standard is at least 30, but 50 is the ideal, regardless of your skin type.

Tans fade, damage stays

Tan fades as cells move upwards and shed off. Tan is never a good thing – it is a sign that your skin is damaged to a certain extent. However, if your tan fades quickly, this is a sign that your skin proliferates (exfoliates) well, which means that beyond the damage you are causing to your skin by tanning, the overall health of your skin is quite good.

Even though a tan has faded, it has still damaged the skin as UV rays can damage the DNA of the 'mother' cell. If a damaged cell divides to make a new cell, that new cell will also be damaged.

To simplify it, tans are bad. When your tan fades, the damage is still there – just bloody protect yourself from the sun, ALL RIGHT! No tan, no 'freckles' and definitely no sunburn. Fake it – I adore a brand called TanOrganic. It's full of skin-friendly ingredients and doesn't dry out the skin.

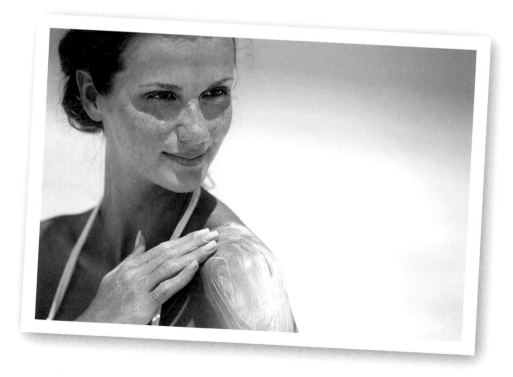

Skin and the Sun

There are many myths involving the effect of the sun on the skin, probably wishful thinking as people love the sun and want to justify being out in it. One of the big ones is that the sun can help and heal acne and congestion. I think from my tone you already know that this isn't true. The sun can temporarily improve the appearance of acne, as UV radiation can subdue how our immune system works which means that the inflammation that causes acne to appear red and swollen won't occur. On top of that, if you're not using sunscreen in the hopes that it'll improve your acne, you'll be tanning so the colour of spots will blend in closer to your new darker skin tone.

The sun does nothing to help with the root of congestion – you'll actually be creating more oil due to associated skin dehydration which will make the problem worse. Your skin will be much better in the long run if you skip the sun and make sure to use your sunscreen.

If you're an oilier and more spot-prone person, you are probably well aware that sweating can bring up more spots, even though many argue that this isn't technically true. I find myself that I will break out in tiny bumps when I'm sweating, especially if I'm using heavier products. Don't cloak yourself in lots of heavy makeup and thick products if you know it's warm out. Keep it light and use products that won't sit on the skin, this will help you to avoid sweat-related spots.

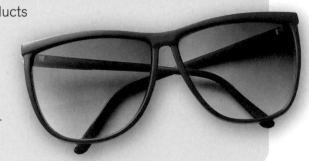

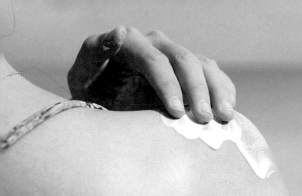

Nothing spoils a holiday like heat rash. It's itchy, it's uncomfortable and some may say it's unsightly. Technically named miliaria, heat rash is what happens when your sweat glands become obstructed and so sweat becomes trapped in the skin, causing inflammation in the form of a rash or rashes across the skin.

It seems like bad advice to simply tell someone not to sweat but really, what you're trying to do with heat rash is sweat as little as possible as this just irritates the rash further. Cotton is your friend – wear light cotton clothes as they let the heat out. Stay hydrated and run cold water on yourself if you're feeling too hot. Stick to mineral sunscreens as sunscreens that use primarily or predominantly chemical sunblocks trap more heat in the skin. Think about it – chemical filters work by absorbing the UV rays so all of that heat gets trapped there, causing heat rash. Use an ice pack on your heat rash to cool it down and help to bring down inflammation.

Sun exposure can cause pigmentation and acids like glycolic acid, lactic acid, azelaic acid and salicylic acid can make your skin more sensitive to light, meaning you could be more susceptible to hyperpigmentation, hypopigmentation and other skin concerns associated with the sun. If the weather is tropical or if you're going on a sun holiday, ditch your acids for a while.

When you're going on holidays or will be exposed to heated sunlight (AKA UVB rays), protect yourself properly. You wouldn't go into battle without a shield, would you? Invest in a very big hat, a good body sunscreen that you know you won't mind wearing and topping up – a sticky, heavy one will put you off applying it – and a facial sunscreen that you can wear under makeup. Opt for a mineral body sunscreen if you are sensitive to chemical sunscreens or prone to heat rash – these sunscreens will usually use zinc oxide and titanium dioxide as their main active ingredients.

If the worst does happen and you do become sunburnt, the most important advice is to not rub oils and thick creams all over it (this includes petroleum jelly) as this traps the heat in the skin. I don't know where people got this idea from but it is not the same as using an after-sun product.

You need to allow the heat to escape for at least the first 24 hours. Pure aloe vera is soothing and will help to reduce the soreness of

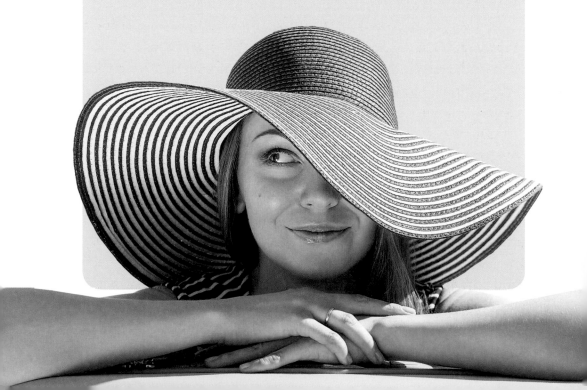

the burn so you are okay to apply this or a specific sensitive after-sun lotion. You have to treat sunscreen as you would a burn.

Avoid a chemical sunscreen the next day and opt for a mineral one instead, as the chemicals may irritate the skin further. You should be in the shade until you are fully healed whenever possible.

If you have blistered, put a plaster on the blistered patch to allow it to heal and prevent it from becoming further damaged – do NOT pop it, touch it, poke at it or leave it exposed to more sun. Really. Sunburn is a big deal and thus should be treated as such.

Don't forget to look after your lips in the sun. How many people worldwide have just forgotten that their lips have skin and allowed them to get burnt? Millions. It is by far the worst type of trout pout.

Accelerated collagen degradation versus collagen degradation

Collagen degradation is the normal breakdown of proteins whereas accelerated collagen degradation means the proteins are breaking down too fast. This is what happens when people age faster. All signs of ageing happen sooner, whether that's a 'drop' in skin (sagging around the eyes and jowls), or lines and wrinkles developing more quickly.

If accelerated collagen degradation is an issue for you, you may also be more prone to redness. To break it down into basics, collagen and elastin degradation happens because enzymes called matrix metalloproteinase enzymes (mouthful, I know, let's just call them MMPs), specifically collagenase and elastase. These enzymes naturally become more active as we age and start to lose the MMP inhibitors that stop them from acting. Our MMP inhibitors are like a teacher in a primary school who stops the rowdy children from getting out and destroying (degrading) the school's grounds. Without the teachers, there would be bits of broken doors and pencils flying everywhere.

However, exposure to sunlight triggers a blast of MMP enzymes even hours after you've been out in the sun. Tobacco prompts MMP enzymes too, which is one of the many, many reasons that smokers age more quickly than non-smokers.

So, our collagen degrades anyway because of the teacher-rowdy-student dynamic that breaks down over time. The older the teacher gets, the less able they are to hold off those rowdy students. However, we can accelerate the process by having a lifestyle that enables more MMP enzymes to be made.

Collagen Degradation FAQs

What is healthy and what is too fast in terms of collagen degradation?

There's no defined rate: it comes down to our DNA. It is a pattern passed down from our parents that can be affected by our choices in life. Sounds scary? Yeah, it kind of is, really.

What if they break down too slowly?

You will live forever! Not really. However, you will look younger for longer. If you keep your MMP inhibitors further into life and refrain from allowing too many MMPs to be triggered, then, technically, your collagen and elastin will remain youthful and you will have fewer lines, wrinkles and your skin will be plumper and more structured and taut.

It's not all bad ...

Collagen degradation sounds negative, but it's normal. Humans are built to degrade over time. I hate to get existential in a book about skin, but it is an inevitable fact.

Ultimately, ageing is a gift. We can fight accelerated degradation of collagen but we can't actually stop it. We can attempt to slow it down, we can load up on Vitamin C to help with our synthesis, we can slather ourselves in rice peptides galore (in studies, rice peptides are shown to aid in the process of stopping MMPs in their tracks), but it will be occurring at one rate or another.

Collagen degradation is natural and cannot be stopped. But accelerated collagen degradation can be helped with by using SPF daily and not over-exfoliating, which is often something we learn the hard way, as well as ensuring you get lots of protein (through food), and Vitamins A and C in topical skincare.

How to Figure Out Your Skin Situation

Before we explore different skin regimes, discuss recommended products and analyse advice and treatments for skin concerns, we need to figure out what your skin is doing right now. And the best way to do this is to take a long hard look in the mirror. I know, I know – this does not sound fun AT ALL. But you know your skin, you know how it looks in the morning and at four o'clock in the afternoon. And you know what you're unhappy with or worried about. So worry not, this is all about helping you.

1. Cleanse your face and don't apply any products.

2. Return to your mirror one hour later. This will ensure that all natural oils are now present in the skin and we can truly decipher your skin and not the residue of the products you use.

3. Touch your T-zone (nose and forehead area). Is there a slip to it? If yes, you are oily. Salicylic cleansers here will be best.

4. Is your T-zone rough? If yes, your skin is dry. In this case you need EFAs to lock in moisture and potentially a glycolic exfoliator twice a week with SPF.

5. Is it tight? If yes, your skin is dry. More EFAs.

6. Does it feel lumpy and bumpy anywhere? If yes, you have excess and trapped oil; salicylic acid is your new best friend.

7. Is it smooth to touch? If yes, you are normal-skinned. Congrats! But don't do nothing. Prevent damage and pump with antioxidants and SPF.

8. Does your face have a shine throughout the day? If yes, you are oily. Wear powder oil-free makeup. (Interesting fact: oil makeup is made to sit on skin that is cooler than 37°C, so makeup in general is not always designed with body heat in mind and will slide more so if oily.)

9. Does any makeup clump or coagulate midday? If yes, you are dry or dehydrated.

10. Can your skin feel tight during the day? If yes, you are dry or dehydrated, try hyaluronic acid in a serum (I love Pestle + Mortar).

11. Are your pores small or large? Are they visible more so on your nose than on your cheeks? If they are small and tight, you are dry-skinned. If large, you are oily. If they are normal, you probably won't really see them at all – your skin will look smooth and your pores will look like tiny pinpricks.

12. Is your skin red? Is it sensitive to touch? Does it always react to new ingredients? Is this a new occurrence? If you answered 'yes' to all of these, your skin is possibly sensitised. We treat sensitised and sensitive skin in much the same way, but with sensitisation, there needs to be a focus on rebuilding the barrier and care taken not to damage or strip it further. We do this by relaxing on the acids for a while until the skin recovers, balancing the skin's pH and providing it with a means to rebalancing its bacteria (e.g. by using probiotic skincare). All of these things can also benefit sensitive skin.

13. To check in on your collagen degradation, look at your peers. If you are more lined or have thinner or more lax skin than your peers who wear sunscreen, don't smoke, don't drink as much and eat well, that's a key sign of accelerated ageing. However, if you are seeing fine lines and 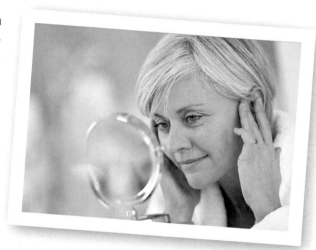 wrinkles from your late thirties onwards, this could very well be normal for you. Look at photographs of older family members about the same age, does your skin look in the same nick? Then it may genuinely be chronological … EMBRACE IT.

14. Dehydrated skin will respond well to water-based hydrators, such as hyaluronic acid. You can still be oily if you are dehydrated, but you won't be if you're truly dry (unless you're combination). Has your skin ALWAYS been dry? Then that is probably your skin type. Dehydration is easily recognisable as your skin will feel taut after a shower. I always distinguish it as it has a slight sheen to it, feels rougher to touch, it puckers if you run your forefinger along it and it laps up product. It is the most common skin condition as most of us don't eat enough EFAs, nor do we drink enough water. We also sit in air-conditioned and centrally heated rooms. Dehydration is easily corrected short term with sheet masks, but, in the longer term, we need fats and oils in our diets and topical skincare.

15. I have yet to meet a person who doesn't have some kind of pigmentation so don't beat yourself up about it. If you stand in front of the mirror and look at the skin around your breasts – where it's unlikely that you'd have any pigmentation unless you're a topless sun worshipper – and chart your skin up towards your décolletage and neck, you will perhaps see some redness on the décolletage. The colour of your neck should be similar to your breasts. Then, on your face you'll see freckles (remember they're only freckles if you're born with them, otherwise they're pigmentation usually from sun exposure) and some discolouration or blotchiness (that may not be too obvious) across your cheeks, usually with more 'freckles' around the hairline. It's good to be aware of your pigmentation but don't panic about it – or anything in this list! It can all be helped.

16. Finally, you want to look at your skin with your spot lens on. If you get spots around your chin, it's usually hormone related. I personally believe spots on the forehead are connected to digestion. If you have spots where your highlighter/bronzer would go, this is usually because your makeup brushes aren't being cleaned properly. Spots around your ears are usually because of your mobile phone. Spots under the skin (i.e. congestion that never materialises into a traditional spot) is usually due to a lack of exfoliation in that area. The biggest mistake people make when identifying spots is

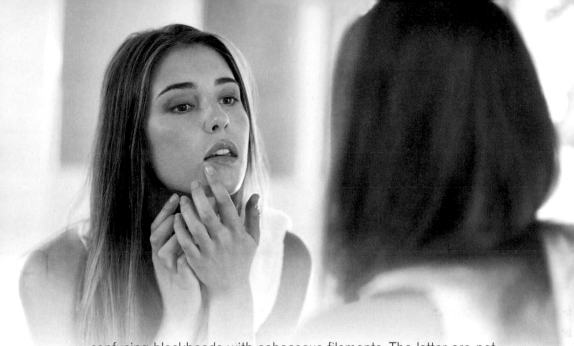

confusing blackheads with sebaceous filaments. The latter are not bad. They are something we all have and they are flat and tiny and if you squeeze them a little worm of oil will come out, whereas if you squeeze a blackhead a thick plug of fat/oil will emerge. A blackhead will have a flat, sometimes slightly raised black circumference. We want to reduce blackheads (never by popping though) whereas sebaceous filaments are our friends. The skin needs oil, remember.

What to Do Now?

Next, it is best to decipher which combination you have (as there may be a few of the aforementioned factors at play) and write them down. Then write beside them which ones affect you the most – like a priority shopping list. For example:

Dehydrated: 3

Lines: 2

Open pores: 1

Then, know that open pores are treated long term as are lines so they may be 1, 2 but 3 is an easier fix so we can remove this and concentrate on 1 and 2.

The Difference Between Women and Men's Skin

Physiologically, men's skin is 25 per cent thicker than women's skin. Men also have more collagen than women and a different composition of connective tissues. Lucky little so-and-so's. These are positives for the most part! The thickness of men's skin means that they visibly age slightly more slowly than women but it also means that it is more difficult for products to penetrate their skin as deeply. Because of this, men can typically handle glycolic acid better.

Hormones also play a role here. Men have more testosterone, which leads to sebaceous glands that work a little harder so men tend to be oilier in nature. This oiliness makes many men prone to blackheads and spots. Have you ever looked up close at the nose of a man who doesn't cleanse? It is like a blackhead strawberry.

I disagree that men cannot see results when using the same skincare as women. The key skingredients remain the same. Men's skin – all skin – needs Vitamin A, antioxidants, sunscreen, EFAs and whatever else is required to treat specific issues.

Thus, men-targeted brands and range are essentially appealing to men through their marketing techniques, the slate-grey packaging, and scents like sandalwood and gun smoke. I might shock you by saying I don't necessarily think this is a bad thing. In an ideal world, the same packaging would appear delightful to us all but, unfortunately, this is far from the truth. If slapping the same solution into a grey bottle gets men to look after their skin, I'm all for it.

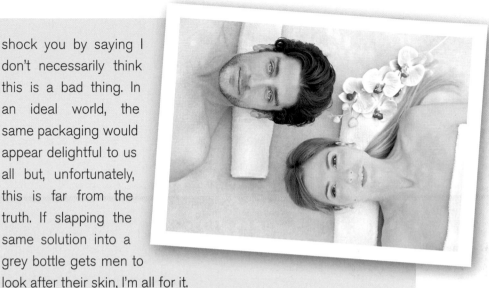

What is an issue is that men's products often contain astringent, stripping, sensitising ingredients, such as harsh perfume ingredients and alcohol. Obviously, these things are just as bad for men's skin as they are for women's skin so we want to exclude them from skincare routines.

Not all men's skincare is the same. Some brands come up with truly innovative products that will actually get men on board. I've seen shaving balms that double as moisturisers – obviously, I'm talking about those without drying alcohols and fragrances but with energising caffeine or peptides – to improve the actual appearance and health of the skin. I've seen cleansers being marketed as cleanser/shower gel duos – the trick is that most cleansers can be used as shower gels in the first place.

To summarise, men need to look after their skin in essentially the same way as women do and I don't mind how they do that one bit – as usual, their skincare routine should be ingredient-led.

Skin Diary Check-in:

Ask yourself the questions about your skin in this chapter and note the responses. You might find that some areas of your skin are oily and others are dry, etc.

You will have gone forensic on your skin for this section so my parting advice is not to obsess over things you didn't quite see before. We all have various combinations of skin concerns, some more prominent than others, but we will all work towards skin health.

Acne

As acne is such a major concern for my clients that it deserves its own chapter, so that you can jump right to it in times of need.

Acne, as I touched on in the Introduction and the Your Mindset chapter, can cause serious issues with confidence – it certainly has for me. It is stigmatised perhaps more than any other skin condition, and, while my goal is to help you get your acne under control, it's also my goal that we stop thinking of acne as an indicator of poor hygiene or that those with perfectly clear skin are in some way superior to those who deal with chronic breakouts. These connotations add to the stress associated with acne and, as we now know, stress will only make things worse.

Acne of all kinds is a skin condition.

Many believe that acne is just something that teenagers get: those sore, swollen, red spots with white-filled tips or the carbuncle-type masses on cheeks. This is acne for sure, but it is more severe. The truth is, everything from tiny skin-coloured bumps and blackheads to red, painful cysts count as acne. Sorry – it's not what you want to hear, but I promised you no BS.

The difference between acne and the odd spot? There really isn't one, but acne can be chronic, persistent and resistant to different forms of treatment. It is when the infection begins to spread deeper into the skin that usually makes the difference between the odd spot and chronic acne.

Note: not every spot is infected. Infected spots happen because of bacteria, such as p. acnes. You'll know if a spot is infected because it will be red, even just in a circle around the spot itself, swollen and, sometimes, tender.

Acne of any form is caused by a build-up of dead skin cells in the pore, the tiny holes you find across the vast majority of your body. This build-up is caused by four potential factors: hormones, hyperkeratinisation (the skin's inability to self-exfoliate), over-production of sebum and the fact that it is a thicker consistency, and, finally, bacteria.

As cells move up through the epidermis, they mature and change. This is what is known as keratinisation. Cells are shed off the skin in a process known as desquamation. However, if this natural exfoliation process is struggling – it starts to slow down after the age of twenty-five – they may become trapped in the pore along with sebum and perhaps bits of cosmetic makeup, causing a plug that forms a spot.

This happens with all spots – the changes that make them bigger and more painful are down to the introduction of bacteria, the health of the cell walls, etc. They are all caused by dead skin cells and sebum that has become trapped in the pore.

Hormones, such as androgens – specifically testosterone (a male sex hormone that is also present in women but usually in smaller doses), fluctuate throughout the menstrual cycle. Hence, it is fairly normal for hormone levels to fluctuate in women and men.

It is androgens that influence our sebaceous glands, telling them how much oil to produce. If we have heightened levels of androgens, such as testosterone, this means that our glands may overproduce sebum, leaving plenty around in our skin cells to become clogged up alongside dead skin cells.

There are other reasons our skin may overproduce sebum. If we strip our skin of its oils through over-exfoliation, our skin may try to compensate by overproducing sebum to keep the skin from becoming dry. All the more reason to say, in the words of TLC, 'No Scrubs'.

Bacteria isn't usually the cause of acne, it is the clogging of the pores that is the cause, but more severe forms are influenced by the p. acnes bacteria getting into the pore and causing infection. This bacteria is responsible for inflammation deep in the pore as it grows rapidly and causes cellular damage. It has very little to do with hygiene but that doesn't mean you shouldn't wash your face.

P. acnes exists on our skin naturally. It is not random old bacteria floating about in the atmosphere. However, if you do pick at acne, then you do risk random old bacteria getting in too.

Blackheads and open comedones (blackheads without a covering of skin or a head) are pretty much just the plug. So how does a spot become more than just these tiny flat plugs? As soon as bacteria hits these bad boys, they become inflamed and red and may fill with pus. All spots have the same origin story, in this sense.

It can also affect the health of the cells that make up the wall of the pore. The health of the pore's walls is really important when it comes to the distinction between different grades of acne (see page 119).

The pore's walls become damaged and rupture, spreading infection deeper and wider and leading to bigger, deeper spots. This is one of the reasons why popping spots is so bad. When you pop spots, you can contribute to the damage of the pore's walls, thus pushing bacteria deeper into the skin. It may seem like a short-term solution but, really, you're making things worse in the long term. I do appreciate it is a fabulous feeling – bra off, Saturday night car crash TV and popping a spot all equals a divine night in. But it is just spreading the bacteria.

Spot Quick Fixes and Remedies

- Avoid wearing cosmetic makeup, especially heavy makeup. A full coverage foundation may seem like the solution to your problem but it is absolutely not. Not only does cosmetic foundation trap sebum and skin cells in the pore as it cannot move past the makeup sitting inside the pore, it can also make lumpier, larger spots more noticeable rather than less. Give your skin a break from the cake and lower the chances of them getting bigger. Mineral (not mineralised) makeup is the way to go.

- Cleanse with salicylic acid-based products. Salicylic acid is a BHA (beta-hydroxy acid) that gently chemically exfoliates the skin, getting rid of the very same dead skin cells that become trapped in the pore causing a spot. It also soothes the skin, brings down redness and inflammation and dries out the spot. Environ B-Active Sebuwash contains tea tree oil and salicylic acid and works wonders on oily and acne-prone skin. It smells fab too!

- Avoid using things that can introduce additional bacteria to the skin or disinfect them. This includes, but is not limited to, phones and makeup brushes. You can apply your makeup with fingers that have been washed with antibacterial soap and you can cleanse with clean hands (or a hyper-clean Cleanse Off Mitt®). You may continue using your phone, though, you might need that. However, give it a wipe with phone-safe, antibacterial wipes. These are the only wipes I will ever own.

- Do not pop your spots. Popping spots, especially if they are not 'ready', causes scabbing, inflammation and infection, and spreads bacteria, causing more breakouts and keeping you in a constant cycle. Popping your acne can also affect your skin in the long term, as in you could be left with permanent scarring and semi-permanent pigment marks. But if you must do it, clean beforehand and treat it as a wound afterwards.

- If you have a big, pus-filled, white pustule (i.e. the head is very clearly visible under a translucent layer of skin) and you really cannot bear being seen with it, you can go ahead and pop it – and this is the only time you should ever pop a spot. The objective is to release the infection. Be careful not to draw blood and to sanitise your hands and your skin carefully with anti-bacterial soap and/or hand sanitiser if you are going to do this.

- Zap the suckers with a spot treatment that includes salicylic acid, lactic acid or even peptides like in Acne Out Active Lotion. Treating the spot this way may cause it to become a little bit corn-flakey around the edges but if you are able to trade that off against size and redness, go for it!

- WEAR YOUR SPF! You should be wearing it every day anyway, that's a given. However, the sun can brand you with acne marks if you do not wear SPF, as acne marks are pigmentation. The area that is discoloured is more likely to mark is not protected. Avène has mattifying, mineral and oil-free options.

- If you have an acne cyst, nodule or a particularly vicious pustule that's causing you pain, hold ice wrapped in a clean piece of tissue or cloth over it for a while. Ice can bring down the inflammation, even if only temporarily. Avoid touching it with your fingers as they are dirty.

- Slather scabs or healing spots in Colostrum Gel to help it heal. Yon-Ka's Hydra No°1 Masque is also great as a spot treatment to speed up healing as is their Serum Vital. Acne Out Lotion and Murad On The Spot lotion are other options.

P. Acnes and Sebum

I find it helpful to understand how P. acnes and sebum work together.

On the top layer of our skin, we all have a bacteria named p. acnes (propionibacterium acnes). Its function is to meet with the oil and form the acid mantle (i.e. the naturally occurring protective layer). The reality is that because of various factors, such as diet or hormonal changes, the skin is not exfoliating itself regularly, so the oil inside the gland whose role it is to secrete out, up and onto the top layer of the skin becomes blocked. The sebum is now trapped inside the skin and becomes enlarged.

P. acnes is a good bacteria desperate to find the sebum to make the protective acid mantle layer, so in he goes to the pore – no invitation, just slips right on in to find his sebum – this is unsolicited and so the body sees it as a foreign object and causes inflammation, which is the redness we see surrounding a spot. The body now sees the p. acnes as a full-on invasion and attempts to expel it.

If the skin is exfoliated and antibacterial options are given to reduce the spot, the spot won't be a problem for more than a few days. But the question is: is this a real solution? And the answer is *no*!

The same scenario is likely to repeat, repeat and repeat until we address the issue about why the sebum (and dead skin cells) are not being released properly. Is it hormone-related? Is it related to an intolerance? Is there a different reason?

Grade 1: Mild

- Grade 1 acne can be called flat acne or non-inflammatory acne as it usually means no redness and no bumps. Blackheads and open comedones are a sign of grade 1 acne and occur because of excess oiliness.

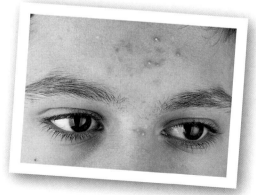

- This type of acne usually doesn't require intense treatment as it may never progress past this point. However, it is important to watch to see if the condition worsens regardless of this.
- Grade 1 acne is most commonly found in the T-Zone (nose and forehead).

Grade 2: Moderate

- With moderate acne, you will have more blemishes like whiteheads (closed comedones) with some inflammation. This is where you may see papules, the type of spot that is small and headless, and even some pustules, the type that are larger and will usually grow a yellow or white head. The whitehead of pustules is made up of white blood cells and sebum mixed with debris.
- Grade 2 usually affects the T-Zone and the cheeks, chin and jaw.

Grade 3: Severe

- Grade 3 means that the papules (red spots) and pustules (white-headed, infected spots) occur in larger numbers and are more visibly inflamed (i.e. larger, redder and more painful).

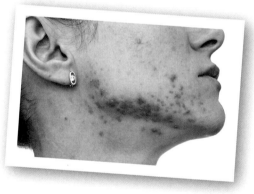

- Spots may join together. Because of this, an area of the skin is infected rather than a single pore. The structure of the skin is compromised because of the collapsing pores and scarring can occur.
- The infection has spread deeper into the skin. A doctor's advice is needed.

Grade 4: Cystic

- Cystic acne is very angry, severe acne. It is deep, very painful and usually over 5 mm in diameter.

- Spots usually have a smooth texture and are very tender. You may also have nodules, which are solid and sore bumps that do not contain pus.
- They can last for absolutely ages and even when they do go away, they can lie dormant before returning. A doctor's advice is needed.

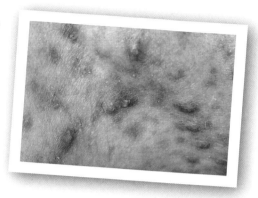

Hormonal Acne

All acne is hormonal. However, women who experience hormonal acne usually find it gets worse during different points of their menstrual cycle (i.e. during their period, or when they're ovulating). It is said that hormonal acne is more likely to happen on the lower half of the face, below your cheekbones, along your jawline, on your chin and around your mouth.

Women who suffer from uterine or ovarian conditions, such as polycystic ovaries and endometriosis, often also suffer from persistent, unresponsive acne, specifically at times when their other symptoms are worse.

Men may experience hormonal acne if they have a hormonal imbalance. Anabolic steroids, which some people take to help to build muscle mass quickly, are synthetic testosterone so they can also cause acne.

Hormonal acne should be treated the same way topically that other acne is treated. For all intents and purposes, it is influenced by the same hormones, such as testosterone and progesterone, even if it is in differing levels.

Acne is more likely to crop up out of nowhere in times when your hormone levels are fluctuating greatly, which is why women who have never had a spot will suddenly get a lot of them during pregnancy or throughout the menopause.

The same goes for times of stress – again, it's the hormones. While I know how upsetting it can be, it will pass. Again, focus on your stress-reducing efforts and mindfulness during more intense times of life.

Bacne

Yep, back acne is now more commonly referred to as bacne. Bacne happens because your back also has sebaceous glands, creating sebum. When you think about it, it's even more difficult for your back to secrete this sebum without it becoming trapped as you are (near) constantly wearing clothes on it. I'd love to see what bacne is like in a nudist colony.

One reason that people get bacne without getting facial acne may be that they are neglecting to prevent acne on their back or to help it. People may be able to keep bacteria at bay on their face enough to prevent facial breakouts whilst using their regular cleanser but many shower gels actually don't contain antibacterial ingredients, such as your typical, fruity, scented, luxurious ones. Bin these! They don't clean; they strip. Dr Bronner is a winner as is Urban Veda when it comes to shower gel brands. Sweat collects on the back, as does bacteria from clothes. Friction from wearing backpacks might also irritate the skin, as may some laundry detergents or fabric softeners. In these cases, it's important to make sure you're washing your clothes enough and not leaving sweat to irritate your skin after you have worked out.

This is also true of bum acne which many find to be exacerbated by non-breathable underwear, such as thongs and the sexy like – it should be cotton all the way, granny pants are to stay.

If you sweat intensely (i.e. on a hot day, during physical exertion), wash yourself with something antibacterial as soon as possible. Shower straight after exercise, those twenty minutes it takes you to get home may be causing the problem. I cover a body brush with a Cleanse Off Mitt® and cleanse my back in the shower the same way I would cleanse my face.

Something people forget about is the effect that shampoo and conditioner can have on your skin. While I'm no haircare professional, I do recommend ensuring that all of the product is thoroughly rinsed from your skin and if you feel your shampoo or conditioner is affecting your skin, avoid any product that contains sulphates, which can reside in the skin and exacerbate the issue. There are plenty of affordable shampoo brands that don't contain this stripping ingredient.

Adult Acne

Having acne in your teenage years is difficult but, perhaps, more expected; it's when most people will get it. Having acne as an adult is arguably more difficult as acne is a stigmatised condition. Many believe that acne occurs due to high sugar intake or not washing yourself, but anyone who has suffered from acne as an adult knows that neither of these are true. Adult acne means that a systemic problem is occurring.

After their teen years, most people find that their hormone levels settle and they stop getting regular spots. This is the norm, so to speak. If you are still getting teenage-level spots as an adult, it is a sign of something else going on.

If you have adult acne, it will be one of two types: continuing acne (meaning that it has carried on from acne that you had in your teenage years without going away) or adult-onset acne (meaning that it begins suddenly when you are an Official Honest-to-God Adult, AKA past the age of twenty-five – in terms of adult acne, as we are all still kids at heart).

Technically, even getting blackheads, bumpiness or the odd two or three spots means that you have acne – it doesn't have to be severe to be chronic. Acne is a medical issue – do not self-diagnose.

There are a few things at play with adult acne:

- **Hormones**: It's nearly misleading to separate acne from hormonal acne as in our experience, the majority of our clients tend to relate their breakouts to hormonal changes. Hormonal imbalances of any scale can cause breakouts, so you may be more likely to have spots during your period, while you are pregnant, while you are on birth control or during the menopause. Clients we've had with polycystic ovaries seem to be more likely to suffer with congestion. If you believe your acne to be hormonal, visit your GP who will run tests and prescribe what they think will help you.

- **Genetic predisposition**: You are more likely to be an acne sufferer if it runs in your family. However, there's not a lot known about why. There are definitely correlations when it comes to adult acne but nobody is quite certain on a lot of things. As a parent, watch out for it as your child reaches their teenage years.

- **Stress**: I personally believe stress is hugely responsible for why adults get acne. Your body responds to stress by bumping up the production of androgens in the body. These androgens stimulate oil glands, leading to extra oil being produced and, therefore, more blackheads, papules and pustules form on the skin. Quit the job. Cancel the mortgage. Live responsibility-free … No?! I didn't think so!

- **Products**: It doesn't matter if products are expensive or cheap – what matters is that they are non-comedogenic. This means that they will not clog the pore – this goes for makeup and skincare. If you are using products without antibacterial ingredients, they probably are not doing a lot for your skin.

- **Dietary intolerances**: I recently had a client who was trying everything to cure their acne – they had even had hormone and blood tests, and they had been on all the products and medications that should help it at some point. This person was particular about what they ate and every day. For lunch they had the same thing: cucumber, brown bread and chicken. People don't have a lot of faith in taking intolerance tests but this person had no other option at this point, and so they gave it a go. Their results came back that saying that they had intolerances to chicken, cucumber and some of the ingredients of brown bread and, within two weeks of removing these foods from their diet, their skin went from grade 4 acne (cystic acne) to grade 2/3 (papules and pustules). So don't count it out!

- **Sugar**: Technically, the jury is still out on this one. Sugar raises insulin levels, which may trigger male hormones and thus increases oil production. However, many dermatologists believe that sugar has no effect on acne.

Ayurvedic Face Mapping

I love Ayurvedic face mapping for acne. I'm all for the newy-newest of skin-related technology. Apply radio-frequency on moi, pummel ultrasound down into the depths of my facial muscles, enhance my skincare to work with my genetic makeup. Do not, however, forget about the ancient traditions of beauty, the concepts and modalities that laid the groundwork for the beauty industry that we know and love today.

Ayurveda is a form of traditional medicine that comes from India that centres around the balance between mind, body and soul. In Ayurveda, people fit into three body categories: vata, pitta and kapha. Vata is the creative, energetic type, prone to restlessness, associated with dry skin. Pitta is the logical, ambitious type but can have a hot temper, associated with sensitive skin. Kapha is the loving type but can be prone to insecurity, associated with oilier skin.

Ayurvedic face mapping is a practice where areas of the face are associated with different body parts and systems. Ayurvedic face mapping is thought to allow you to see how your body as a whole is affecting skin concerns – it gives you a bigger picture on the skin that perhaps you may not see if you're focusing on the skin as a separate entity.

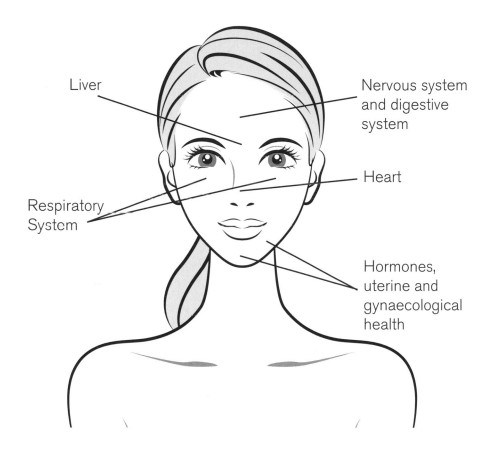

Liver

Nervous system
and digestive
system

Heart

Respiratory
System

Hormones,
uterine and
gynaecological
health

Forehead

Let's start from the top, shall we? In ayurvedic face mapping, your forehead
is connected to the nervous and digestive systems and associated with
the Vata Dosha. If you have breakouts on your forehead, it may suggest
an imbalance in your gut or sluggish bowels, poor circulation and stress
in your general life.

Between your eyebrows

The area between your eyebrows is thought to correspond to your liver so
if you're breaking out here, it may be due to liver problems or a sign that

you should be cutting down on your alcohol consumption. (To be clear – we are not referring to medical problems here.)

Nose

In Ayurveda, the nose is associated with the heart. If you have breakouts or redness in the nose, it is supposed that it may be caused by problems with circulation or blood pressure.

Cheeks

The cheeks are connected to your respiratory system, so those who have problems breathing and with their lungs may see breakouts or skin concerns in this area. Are you a smoker with problems in this area?

Chin and jaw

This is believed to be correlated to hormones and uterine and gynaecological health, or bacterial overgrowth in your gut (probiotics, what what?!). If you suffer from a hormonal imbalance, this is where you may see congestion.

Do I believe we can treat the skin on the basis of ayurvedic face mapping alone? No. Am I suggesting that just because you get spots on your cheeks you have respiratory problems? Also no … Maybe you just need to wipe down your phone the odd time.

I do believe that it is a helpful mode of secondary or tertiary skin analysis. If something just isn't adding up with regard to your own skin concerns, it may be helpful to think about the ayurvedic correlations.

Treating Acne

Treating acne requires treating a few different aspects. You're looking to bring down inflammation and redness, clear out the pores, control sebum production, hydrate the skin, and prevent and lighten pigmentation and scarring.

Acne treatment is a tough nut to crack as it truly depends on each individual's skin. When it comes to mild acne, such as blackheads, open comedones, closed comedones and small, infrequent, non-painful white-heads, a combination of salicylic acid on the outside and natural antiseptic and anti-inflammatory ingredients, like tea tree oil, along with taking phyto-nutrients like DIM, internally can bring it to a halt. Grade 1 and 2 acne can be treated by aestheticians like myself – book yourself a nerdie consult.

Grade 3 and 4 acne needs to be treated by a GP or a dermatologist. There is only so much that topical skincare can tackle and it is not worth it to deny yourself treatment if you're in pain, whether that is physical or emotional. Your GP may prescribe antibiotics, to be taken orally, topically or both.

Another topical treatment for acne is benzoyl peroxide, which is more effective than salicylic acid on nodular or cystic acne. For many, the next step if a course of antibiotics hasn't helped is the hormonal route. Hormonal treatments are most commonly birth control pills like Yaz or Dianette which are proven to help in the control of sebum regulation and acne. These are a medical treatment so the decision to take them should not be made lightly.

The last-resort solution is usually isotretinoin (known primarily as Roaccutane in Europe and Accutane in America). I've been on Roaccutane myself and, let me tell you, it is not something to be taken lightly, and, absolutely, is something that must be monitored by a doctor or dermatologist. It can cause dryness, redness and itching, and can often send your skin in the other direction as it dries up all sebum. It is a fairly extreme medication but the slog is worth it if nothing else has worked for you.

I feel Roaccutane gets a lot of bad press but, for some people, it can really help. It did for me. I noticed huge improvements within three weeks. I advise not Googling that side-effects – thanks for the scaremongering, internet – and going straight to your doctor if you think it's for you. Some people experience side-effects on isotretinoin which is worth noting too. Isotretinoin is a retinoid, meaning it is a form of Vitamin A. The forms we use in cosmeceutical skincare and supplements are much less powerful, which is why isotretinoin is only used as a last resort.

When it comes to reducing inflammation, infection and redness and preventing spots from occurring, I'm obsessed with a supplement called Skin Accumax from Advanced Nutrition Programme, as we've already discussed. It contains Vitamin A which is essential for healthy cell turnover and a phytonutrient known as DIM (diindolylmethane) which has been shown to balance the 'cellular inflammatory response' and helps to balance oestrogen metabolism. It was originally created as a follow-on from the use of Roaccutane as a maintenance step.

I also believe the congestion-prone should be taking omegas too, as omegas help to support the skin's lipid layer and, in turn, ensure that moisture stays within the skin. Dehydration can lead the skin to compensate by overproducing oils. And then you have a vicious cycle on your hands.

In terms of topical treatments, salicylic acid is the acid you're looking for as it speeds up the skin's own proliferation process and gets into the pore to clear out the plug of sebum and dead skin cells.

In my opinion, glycolic acid is not ideal for those who overproduce oil. Glycolic draws everything out and, if your skin is constantly creating these blockages because of excess oil, it will never stop being drawn out.

A salicylic cleanser is usually enough and then you can spot treat using a salicylic-based pad or a peptide spot treatment. Hyaluronic acid (not an exfoliating acid) is a great way to hydrate congestion-prone skin as it is hydric rather than lipidic (water instead of oil). Jump to our skingredients section for more on salicylic, glycolic and hyaluronic acid (see page 214).

Preventing post-inflammatory hyperpigmentation (PIH, acne marks) requires topical Vitamin A and lightening ingredients. Lightening serums, like IMAGE Iluma serum and Neostrata Enlighten serum, contain ingredients including liquorice-root extract and Vitamin C which inhibit the enzyme tyrosinase and stop pigmentation from developing.

When it comes to treating pigmentation after it has already developed, pigmentation lightening spot treatments that contain kojic acid and other lighteners (see page 225) can be beneficial as can regular exfoliation with salicylic acid, lactic or glycolic acid, but, as has been mentioned, not too much.

Obviously, if you are getting lesions, you want them to heal quickly and this is why I recommend Environ's Colostrum Gel to those with acne because colostrum contains growth factors that contribute to the healing rate and health of skin cells. These growth factors send messages to the skin that tell the skin to repair itself and regenerate which makes it fantastic for bringing up the healing time of spots. It also improves the texture of spots and minimises the damage that acne can cause to the skin.

Textural scarring requires stimulation of the dermis, so you're looking at in-salon treatments, specifically micro needling, which I believe to be the most beneficial for acne scarring.

In short, in the long-term fight against acne, whatever the root cause may be, we have:

- salicylic acid to dissolve oil and aid scarring
- Vitamin A to repair and balance oil secretion, skin exfoliation rate, possibility of scarring and skin immunity
- hyaluronic acid to aid water and hydration
- Colostrum Gel to strengthen, soothe and calm
- Skin Accumax supplements containing DIM phytonutrient
- contraceptive pill (this needs a prescription), but won't fix the problem alone in my experience; topical treatments are still advisable
- benzoyl peroxide (this needs a prescription)
- Isotretinoin (a last resort, this needs prescription)
- sunscreen/SPF to shield from further scarring

But don't forget, treating the skin internally is key. We can mop the oil till the cows come home externally, but what we do internally to address the imbalance is key.

Spots FAQs

Why are blackheads black?
Blackheads are black because when the plug is left exposed to oxygen, it oxidises and turns black!

Whiteheads versus blackheads?
A whitehead is a blackhead that has developed skin over it and grown further.

What's the difference between a cyst and a spot?
A cyst is a daddy spot with a circumference the size of Jupiter. Cysts occur because of damage of the pore's walls and spreading of infection and thus more inflammation, hence the redness and pain.

Is popping a spot out of the question?
Popping a spot leads to a spread of bacteria both on the surface

and underneath the skin. It can rupture pore walls and cause long-term damage, scarring and post-inflammatory hyperpigmentation. If it is ripe (i.e. white or yellow 'soft' head), push up from below gently with tissue-wrapped fingers, like making a volcano explode and stop before it bleeds (if it bleeds, you've caused damage). Use antiseptic after to help it heal.

Is a sebaceous filament a spot?
Do you have lots and lots of tiny, greyish or flesh-coloured dots around your nose, between your eyebrows or on your chin? You probably think they are clogged pores or blackheads. Newsflash: they are probably sebaceous filaments.

Sebaceous filaments are just hair follicles that have collected a bit of dead skin and sebum. If you squeeze them, they will emit a tiny greyish or yellowish spiky worm. We don't *want* to squeeze them though as they serve the purpose of helping direct sebum to the surface of the skin. Even if you squeeze them, they are likely to return. Leave them be, they are your friends, not your foes. To minimise their appearance opt for regular exfoliation (again, with acids, not scrubs) and ensure you cleanse properly. If they really, really bother you, you can have them professionally extracted every once in a while. Vitamin A may reduce these also.

Acne Scarring

Cystic and nodular acne (the upper end of grade 3 and grade 4) are the types of acne that most frequently cause scarring. This is because the acne has grown deeply into the skin, too far into the epidermis layer. This damages the skin and tissue that lies beneath and the body will try to heal the damage caused. During this reparation process, the body will produce collagen, the protein that gives the skin its structure. If the wrong type or amount of collagen is produced, a scar can occur (too little collagen will produce a pitted or depressed scar, and too much collagen will cause a raised scar).

Scarring is more likely to occur on areas where acne has not had time to completely heal before a new breakout occurs in the same place. If you do not act fast when you have inflamed acne (grade 3 or 4), you may develop scars. This is why it is important to treat acne rather than cover it with makeup, even though it is easier and cheaper to do the latter.

Acne scars can happen to squeezers, pickers and poppers. You should *not* touch acne that does not have a very obvious, very soft and very white head. Having a set of long nails does not give you a qualification to do your own at-home extraction and you can irreparably damage your skin.

What you can do to prevent and treat acne scarring:

- Treat existing acne to prevent future scarring. Via a consultation, get yourself on an active skincare routine (retinol/salicylic acid-based products).
- Don't pick at spots, pop them or do anything that could damage the tissue.
- If you already have acne scars, micro-needling could help especially after twelve weeks of topical Vitamin A application, in my experience, as this achieves results. Tiny needle tips pierce the skin, penetrating the dermis and stimulating the growth of collagen and elastin. It is through this that micro-needling evens out the texture and tone of acne scars.
- Laser resurfacing (e.g. with the Lumenis machine) tricks the skin into thinking it is being harmed, triggering the uppermost layer to shed off and enabling a new layer of skin to form. This can be effective when it comes to acne scarring, depending on the depth or rise of the scar itself.

- Chemical peels may also help but they are not as effective as micro-needling or laser treatments.

So You Want to Pop That Spot?

Hold on.

You really shouldn't pop spots, not even the tiny little whiteheads that crop up around the edges of your nose, not even 'self-extracting' blackheads with those little metal sticks (you are not a professional and you *will* go too hard at it and possibly cause broken capillaries). Popping any spot may cause post-inflammatory hyperpigmentation and cause a spread of bacteria downwards further into the skin.

However, if you simply cannot bear it and you have a ripe spot (a whitehead with very little skin over it) here is the safest way (not the *safe* way, just the safest) to pop it.

1. Realise you are evacuating an infection.
2. Clean your hands thoroughly with antibacterial soap and hand sanitiser (alcohol-free, if you please, as alcohol dries out the skin).
3. Wrap tissue or cotton pads around your forefingers or wear gloves to keep the skin clean.
4. Use the side of the forefingers to press the skin; do *not* go straight in with the top of your nails.
5. Think of the spot as a volcano (and, yes, it can both look and feel like one sometimes – mine need passports, do yours?!). The

whitehead you see is actually a bank of bacteria underneath in a wider circumference. The head of the spot is only the visible gunk. It is actually spread out further under what you see, so you need to leave room between your fingers to get it all and not just the top of the head.

6. Place two fingers either side of the bulbous spot and press down firmly and outwards away from the spot – this will force the bacteria within to drive upwards and draw a wider amount from underneath out.

7. When the bacteria is eliminated, stop – do not wait for blood as this is asking for scarring.

8. Place an antibacterial solution on it – be aware that it is a wound. You can use the antiseptic cream such as Savlon. I opt for Savlon as it's antibacterial and serves a purpose because you have just created a wound, whereas something like Sudocrem will just soothe the skin.

9. Do not put makeup, etc. directly over it – it is an opening into the skin. Only put makeup on the area when it has healed over. If it is still an open hole on your face, avoid applying even mineral makeup wherever possible. It should heal over quickly enough, as long as you don't knock it off anything or pick at it. Once it's scabbed over it is healing and protected so you can then wear mineral makeup as it won't get in.

10. Be aware that therapists have methods to remove in a professional environment so if it is a regular occurrence do book in for 'lancing'.

11. If you insist on popping a spot, it's best to do it at night before you go to bed so you give it time to repair as you sleep and

you're not covering the wound – which is what it is – with SPF or makeup that will likely contain chemicals.

When everything has calmed down, mineral makeup can help to camouflage without exacerbating. Taking zinc internally will help the inflammation and taking Vitamin C internally will prevent the redness thereafter. And have I ever mentioned Vitamin A?

For some, acne is something that they may be able to reduce through making small lifestyle and skincare changes. For others, they will try everything and really struggle to find a solution, including Roaccutane. People will try all of the medical routes and eventually take dairy out of their diet and see a major difference – be careful here and ensure that you get adequate nutrients if you do go dairy-free yourself (with medical advice). Acne is still very much something that we don't understand 100 per cent as far as skin conditions go, but scientists are working on a vaccine.

Ultimately, while my goal is to help clear up skin, I believe that acne of any kind needs to be normalised and destigmatised. We're not dirty because we have spots and we're not all sugar fiends. Why do we feel so bad about red bumps on our faces? It is an illness like any other illness and you would not make fun of someone with chronic migraines, would you? Fair play to Saoirse Ronan, Kendall Jenner and Lorde for speaking about their experiences. We're all hooman after all.

Skincare

It's time to get down to the business of the best practices in your daily skincare routine, as well as navigating the overwhelming world of skincare products.

In the 1980s and 1990s, large skincare brands taught us a three-step rule: cleanse, tone and moisturise. When I was training with CIDESCO (I subsequently taught this method), we were taught to match cleansers to skin types, that toners are to remove the cleanser and that moisturisers are to hydrate the skin, and should also match the skin's type. Today, this is not a guide that I follow. I don't believe in guiding a skin because of its skin type (as you know), but, instead, I concentrate on the skin's condition, and its current health and needs.

My essential steps for anyone are as follows:

Morning

1. Double-cleanse, including pre-cleanse and treatment cleanse (inactive by day, meaning a non-exfoliating acid base).
2. Apply a serum with Vitamins A, C and, E, antioxidants and peptides.
3. Apply SPF.

Night

1. Double-cleanse, including pre-cleanse and treatment cleanse (inactive and active alternating*).
2. Apply serum, the same as the morning with an odd sprinkle of hyaluronic, radiant serums, etc. as an extra.
3. Apply moisturiser, if you want, but it's not essential. Ideally, your skin makes its own moisture, and will the longer you correct it with the right skingredients.

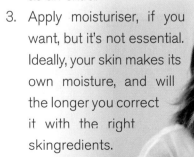

*Active Versus Inactive Cleansing:

Inactive products are soothing, calming and not disrupting, and yet serve a positive purpose beyond smelling nice and cleansing. They are passive and they won't have enzymes or acids in them. 'Active' means it causes physical and enzymatic changes in the skin, so they do more than cleanse, they target lines, wrinkles, skin exfoliation, etc. An example of an active product would be lactic-, glycolic-, polyhydroxy- or salicylic-acid-based cleansers, which we'll explore in more detail shortly.

This is a core daily regime. If you use any more steps than listed above, they should have a justified place in your routine.

Don't use anything just for the sake of it. And nothing purely because it smells nice. Also, be mindful of the fact that you can have too much of certain ingredients. For example, using high amounts of acids in multiple products daily and nightly can be detrimental to your skin – everything should be in moderation.

Let's go through each step in more detail.

Cleanse

The cleansing step is vital, there are no two ways about it. Without any judgement, it surprises me how many people I meet who admit they have never fully understood the importance of it. Cleansing removes the oil, debris and pollution accumulated on the skin after a long, hard day. It removes any dust particles and oil secretion and clears skin cell blockages in the morning. Without cleansing, the remaining products that are then applied will not penetrate evenly. Often people who don't wear makeup feel there is no need for them to cleanse – but unless you live in a secluded cave, there is!

The concept of double-cleansing is key – it is a practice that therapists have been doing for years. It's referred to as a trend in women's magazines, but double cleansing is the ideal practice for skin health. Simply put, you wash/clean your face twice within the same session.

Pre-cleanse

Ideally, a pre-cleanser is an oilier-based product with a balmy consistency that enables the oil be removed thoroughly. Remember, oil cuts through oil. Oilier-skinned hoomans may panic at the thought of an oil-based solution on their face and be fearful that more oil will add to their problems – there is an element of truth to this if the oil is not removed thoroughly – however, oil will break down oil. Simple as. Arguably, it's more needed in an oilier skin! Also makeup wearers will most likely have oily residue from their products and this needs to be dissolved.

My ideal pre-cleanser is my own product, the Cleanse Off Mitt®. Little plug there, but it is fantastic. The reason it works is that the microfibre, which the Cleanse Off Mitt® is made of, removes makeup when it is wet. When skin is covered in oils and makeup, it has a negative charge and

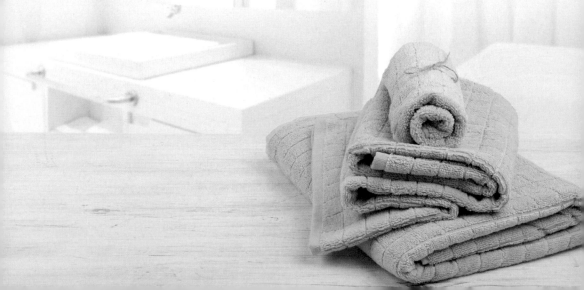

the microfibre when wet has a positive charge. As you remember from science class, opposites attract.

If you're using a microfibre pre-cleansing tool, wet it, wring it out and rub it across your face very gently either outwards and downwards or in small circular motions. Follow it up with your cleanser to achieve your double-cleanse.

If you're using a pre-cleansing balm, oil or fluid, massage this thoroughly into your skin. Amounts may vary but your face should be slick with it. Make sure it makes a multicoloured globby mess and then remove it thoroughly with a warm face cloth (or the Cleanse Off Mitt®).

The Skin Nerd approved pre-cleansers:

- Dermalogica PreCleanse Balm

- Yon-Ka Lait Nettoyant

- Environ Dual Action Pre-Cleansing Oil

- natural oils like coconut oil or jojoba oil (so long as they are thoroughly removed afterwards)
- Cleanse Off Mitt® - I'm biased!

The Cleanse Off Mitt® Versus a Face cloth

The Cleanse Off Mitt® has smaller, looped fibres which allow more control and angles to remove debris. It is lighter so there is less drying time and it is more hygienic. Using a Cleanse Off Mitt® to remove your cleanser is optimal as most tend to splash and go which leaves a residue.

Treatment cleanser

The second part of cleansing is a 'treatment cleanser', which is targeted to suit a particular skin type or skin concern (e.g. ageing, pigmentation, redness, oilines, congestion).

The Skin Nerd approved treatment cleansers:

- IMAGE Clear Cell Clarifying Gel Cleanser (active)
- Biofresh Probiotic Cleansing Milk (inactive)
- Gallinée Foaming Facial Cleanser (inactive)
- Neostrata Foaming Glycolic Wash (active)
- Murad AHA/BHA Exfoliating Cleanser (active)
- Environ SkinEssentiA AVST Mild Cleansing Lotion (inactive)

I am a huge fan of using a probiotic cleanser every morning – this is more than a cream cleanser, it adds good bacteria to the skin. Then, at night, I promote acid-based exfoliating cleansers to be used Mondays, Wednesdays and Fridays, with the probiotic cleanser on Tuesdays and Thursday nights also. On the weekend, I would give the acids a break and stick with the probiotic cleanser morning and night. This is an example of inactive/active cleansing. Use your active/exfoliating cleanser every two or three nights, and use your probiotic or other inactive cleanser on the nights in between, as well as every morning. The overall concept is to 'give *and* take', as opposed to just taking.

Exfoliating cleansers enable the exfoliation regime to be part of our cleanser. It removes the need for a separate exfoliator and a traditional toner, and enables the serums that follow to penetrate into the skin evenly. The skin should be exfoliating itself every twenty-eight days but, from the age of twenty-five, it tends to slow down, and so acids encourage this natural process when it needs a helping hand. Over-use will irritate so, like everything in life, use in moderation.

We will drill down further into exfoliating ingredients in the skingredients chapter (see page 213), but, for now here's what you need to know:

- Glycolic-based cleansers are exfoliating in nature and assist the skin in its natural cell turnover process.

- Lactic-acid cleansers and polyhydroxy acid cleansers (PHAs) are a more gentle and effective form of exfoliating.

- Salicylic acid is an acid saved solely for oily, 'under the spots' spots and acne-prone skin as it is oil soluble. IMAGE Clear Cell Clarifying Cleanser contains so much salicylic acid, it's like a skin-friendly power hose that gets into all nooks and crannies and leaves a gentle tingling sensation.

*Tip: Use the inactive cleanser as an eye make-up remover and cleanse thoroughly and follow with the treatment cleanse.

I alternate this when I'm more congested (such as when I'm really stressed) with other less-active cleansers as it is so strong. If you used it too often, your face would be sensitised. I tend to advise using this every second night to start (if you're quite congested) then reduce to every third night, then every fourth when the skin becomes clear and less oily and lumpy. A consultation is key along with a 'check-in' a few weeks on.

It's best to use acid-based cleansers at night as a rule of thumb, as we're not always religious with our SPF during the day (though we should be!) and after you have used an acid cleanser, you need to be mindful of sun exposure.

Choosing the right cleanser for you, outside of ingredients and concerns, is about a texture and feeling that you will like and that will suit your skin. Skincare shouldn't be a chore. For the most part, you can choose between the following types of cleansers:

- **Foaming washes** are predominantly for a resilient skin that can handle a lot. Foaming washes can often be quite stripping. Many people opt for washes even though they no longer need them. It is psychological as perhaps they needed washes in their teen years and love the tight feel of the skin post-wash. This is no longer necessary. Choose with today's skin in mind, so avoid them unless from a cosmeceutically grounded brand, such as Neostrata's Foaming Glycolic Cleanser. Saying that, the aforementioned Gallinée cleanser is a foam but isn't stripping at all, it is actually quite hydrating.

- **Washes** are usually preferred to foams for oily skinned folks who are always told to opt for a foam. They're a tiny bit foamy or bubbly to help draw oil from the skin. Most should be avoided by the severely dry-skinned but they are suitable for use on normal-skinned or oily skinned hoomans. For this kind, I like IMAGE Ageless Cleanser.

- **Cream cleansers**, **milks** and **cleansing lotions** are associated with dry skin and dehydrated skin as they usually don't contain exfoliating ingredients and are more hydrating. On the other hand, they may not be great at getting rid of excess oil. I would usually suggest removing them with water (a wet Cleanse Off Mitt® is ideal) regardless of what the instructions say. These are best for very sensitive skin, very dry skin and mature skin. The Gallinée or Bioactive probiotic cleanser is a good cream cleanser example and the IMAGE Vital C cleanser is another. There are also cleansers to avoid (or at least be mindful of). These include wipes, micellar water and extremely foamy cleansers.

Wipes

By now, you should know that I could write a whole separate book based on my hatred of wipes. Wipes are depended on far too much for ease of time and affordability, yet they are stripping and dehydrating skin. They irritate it even if you don't feel it. They do not clean the skin thoroughly

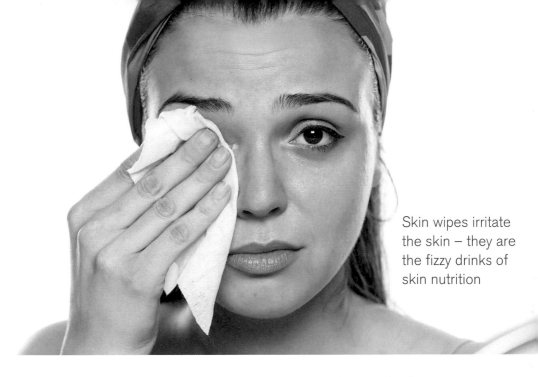

Skin wipes irritate the skin – they are the fizzy drinks of skin nutrition

and they are not a good skin-health decision. I used wipes for fourteen days consecutively and the deterioration in my skin was shocking. I had increased my acne by two grades, which is why I created the Cleanse Off Mitt® – a reusable, convenient alternative to wipes that is kind to your skin. #BinTheWipes – I urge you to join the movement.

Micellar water

Micellar water from authentic French brands or from brands that truly care about skin health is not so bad, as they often do not contain the fragrances and preservatives that strip skin of its oils, or dehydrate and photosensitise skin (AKA make the skin more sensitive to light).

I have been known to call micellar water users glorified wipe users and I believe this is for good reason. Some brands really take the mick with what they consider to be micellar water, to the point that they are essentially liquid wipes. They bulk up their micellar water with drying alcohols, fragrances and harsh preservatives for the purpose of prolonging shelf-life. If you must use it as a pre-cleanser, I approve of Bioderma as it has a lot less alcohol in it (with the pink lid) or Decleor Micellar Water.

One of the issues that I see with micellar water is the same as the one I see with wipes. You are just moving dirt, grime and oils around on your skin. Throughout your day, you are walking through polluted air, touching everything and then touching your face and pumping sebum out to help protect your skin – and all of this builds up. If we do not thoroughly remove this build up, we are asking for congested skin (i.e. blackheads, whiteheads and any other type of spot).

The majority of people who use micellar water are not actually using it as a pre-cleansing step, which would be infinitely better, but as their sole mode of cleansing. Just as with wipes, using micellar water leaves you with an incomplete cleanse and leaves a residue on the skin, (that's like a semi-oily film), meaning that any products applied thereafter may not penetrate properly. You need to be double-cleansing in such a way that your first step removes at least the high 90 per cent of your makeup and any oil and grime that has collected on the surface of your skin so that your second step is removing any build-up of dead skin cells and treating the skin however you please, whether it be with acids, with probiotics or with vitamins.

Extremely foamy cleansers

I'm also wary of overly foamy cleansers where the foam doesn't serve a purpose, as these are unnecessary and often stripping. Foaming cleansers are usually the first cleansers people use in their teenage years and they are packed full of ingredients that make them foam and, usually, nothing else (with the exception of Neostrata

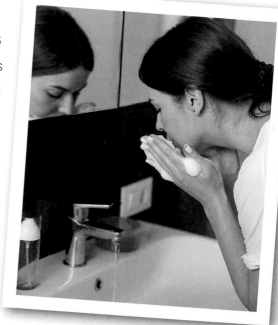

and Gallinée and other foams that actually do something). A key culprit for this type of foaming occurring is a surfactant known as sodium lauryl sulphate, a sulphate that is an irritant especially to sensitive skin. It can cause damage to your skin's barrier and leave it dehydrated and gasping for moisture. If you see this ingredient as one of the first listed on the packaging, avoid the product.

Cleansers that don't truly cleanse or do anything

There are some cheap-as-chips cleansers that contain lovely tea tree oil or Vitamin E or other ingredients that can be added to skincare quite cheaply, but there are others that are, essentially, fatty alcohols mixed with trace amounts of vitamins so they can pop it onto the packaging that it is 'kind to skin, vitamin enriched and alcohol-free'. I see why some want to just clean their face, but you could be hydrating it with a hydrating cleanser or brightening a bit with a brightening cleanser. Why not?

Most active cleansers will be procured after a consultation with a skin therapist but there are some active or cosmeceutical ranges available in pharmacies or online such as Neostrata. If you're looking for a specific active ingredient in a cleanser, such as Vitamin C or salicylic acid, check to see how high it is on the ingredient list. The higher it is, the more of it there is in the product. Buy cleansers from brands that are fairly transparent on their packaging and on their websites about what the ingredients do, whether these brands are cosmeceutical or cosmetic. If a brand tells you that their cleanser 'softens and evens out skin tone', they could be saying pretty much anything. Google the ingredients thoroughly and you'll probably be able to see if they do what they say they do.

Cleansing how-to

Sixty seconds is the ideal time for a thorough cleanse. I opt to wet my hands, pump a two-euro size amount of product into the palm of my hands and then massage upwards (from the nipple up – remember, we treat the neck and décolletage with the same respect that we treat the face). Massage outwards from the nose to support lymphatic drainage and bring down puffiness.

We massage this into a pre-cleansed wet face with freshly washed hands. Sixty seconds is a tough and lengthy process for many, but I encourage breathing properly for this golden minute. See it as essential 'me time' to calm, centre and cleanse. CCC! Breathe in and out calmly and truly take the time to centre and catch up in yourself.

Some people over-cleanse, stripping all of the natural oils from the skin while others do not remove the cleanser thoroughly. Be sure to use a mitt, face cloth or muslin cloth to wash off your cleanser. Ensure the water is warm and not hot. Overuse of hot face cloths cause broken capillaries and dry out the skin – you've been warned.

You can also use the Cleanse Off Mitt® combined with your treatment cleanser if time isn't on your side. Wet your face, massage the mask with treatment cleanser onto your face in nice circular motions and rinse with the same side of the mitt. Then use the other unused side of the mitt to remove any residue. I have a few Cleanse Off Mitts® on the go and wash them each week.

Why removing your makeup at night is essential

Makeup is designed to look pretty. The packaging, the texture, the ease of application and the way it looks on your face is its main goal. The skin-oriented ingredients are less of a priority, which is why I tend to break out when I change my makeup or have blockages on my contour line when I change things up.

The reality of makeup is that the skin is not designed to have anything sit on it for such long periods of time, so it's important to remove these fats, oils and ingredients that are designed for colour and pigment, food and cosmetic dyes which are deemed non-toxic for the skin are not necessarily deemed 'healthy' either. The pollution and oil are also trapped in there in the pores and so we need to remove all of this. I use white towels at home as a way of checking that all my

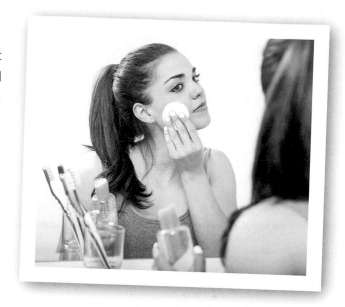

makeup is gone. If you use grey or navy or any other coloured towel, you won't see the black liner and mascara remnants as clearly and may be fooling yourself. You need to remove all traces of everything – as well as the residual cleanser used to take it away – so that the next steps in your routine can work effectively and be absorbed by the skin.

Determined to prove a point, I once went nineteen days wearing my makeup every night and, boy, did my skin suffer. I had more breakouts, congestion was a major issue, my skin became more reactive and, perhaps worst of all, I just didn't feel clean. My bedsheets weren't too happy either. I don't suggest you do the same trial, just take my word for it. You're welcome.

Toner

I tend not to advocate the use of toners. I'm not a fan. I feel the name over-promises and under-delivers! Many toners are alcohol-laced and this can have negative effects on your skin. Not *all* alcohols are bad for the skin, but I've listed on the following page some drying alcohols to avoid, typically found in toners:

- denatured alcohol (also seen as alcohol denat)

- isopropyl alcohol

- SD alcohol

- methanol

- benzyl alcohol

Often, these alcohols are included so that the product dries on to the skin quickly – but fast-drying, when caused by these types of alcohol, is not a good thing. They are also used to help preserve products. These types of alcohol damage the skin's barrier instantaneously and cumulatively, over time, your skin's barrier will no longer be able to help your skin retain moisture or defend itself from things getting in, leading to sensitised, sore skin.

In the short term, toners strip the skin of its natural oils, the very things that keep it healthy, and it is this stripping that leaves the skin feeling 'less oily'. Your skin is no idiot, though, and it may notice this and overproduce oil to compensate, leaving you oilier than you were in the beginning.

Treatment toners are active products with acids in them and serve a purpose. However, if your cleanser already has this ingredient, there is no need to double-dose.

Serum

After a thorough double cleanse, I then opt for serums. Serums are like concentrated moisturisers that can deliver their goodies further into your skin, whereas moisturisers just leave most of them on the surface or in the very uppermost layers of the *stratum corneum*.

Vitamin C-based serums assist with redness, discoloration and work against ageing. Hyaluronic serums provide a drink of moisture to the skin. Antioxidant serums are ideal as they are the protector of skin health. Lightening serums are also ideal and assist clarity and even skin tone.

You'll also find serums with more than one purpose. For example, you'll find Vitamin C and soothing ingredients in lightening serums, and you'll find hyaluronic acid in antioxidant serums and vice versa. Vitamin C itself is a potent lightening agent, an antioxidant and great for ageing. Vitamin A is also key –

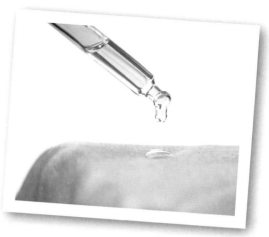

preferably in serum form as it better penetrates the skin.

The Skin Nerd approved serums:

- Environ Skin EssentiA AVST Moisturiser: It calls itself a moisturiser but we consider it a serum in our Nerd World because it is so potent. It absorbs into the skin in a way only a serum could. I love the step-up system of introducing Vitamin A into the skin, as topical Vitamin A is something everyone (bar pregnant hoomans) should be using every day for the rest of their lives.

- Neostrata Enlighten Illuminating Serum: This is fab for those who are pigment prone. It contains soothing tyrosinase inhibiting liquorice root extract, Vitamin C, a brightening peptide and hydrating ingredients too.

- SkinCeuticals C E Ferulic: This bad boy costs an arm and a leg, but it contains real L-ascorbic acid, the purest form of Vitamin C, stabilised for use on the skin as well as Vitamin E and ferulic acid so it is a potent brightener and the best antioxidant protection out there.

- IMAGE Iluma Intense Lightening Serum. This provides general radiance along with antioxidant capabilities.

- Académie Scientifique De Beauté 8h Radiance Serum: gives an instantaneous glow like no other.

Serums are often the priciest part of a good skincare routine, so you really have to know how to apply them. You only need one petit-pois-sized droplet for your forehead and per each cheek. Gently smooth it across and down your skin (all the way down to your nipples) with the tip of your fingers. Scrubbing it or rubbing it in will mean that your fingertips get all of those delicious skingredients. Your face, neck and décollétage need that Vitamin A – your fingers, not so much.

You can mix your serums together. I am a fan of making a serum 'soup' and then applying it all at once. This works better if each serum is of a similar consistency (i.e. creamy and creamy). For example, I would mix Environ AVST and Environ Colostrum Gel, or IMAGE Ormedic Serum and the Neostrata Enlighten Serum.

If you are using more than one, each with its own consistency, I recommend starting with the lightest and moving through to the thickest consistency to enable the products to penetrate. If the thickest serum is applied first it will impede the others from penetrating.

Give it a minute or two to sink into your skin when going to bed, but leave it about five minutes before applying SPF when using in the daytime. Other products can affect how effective your sunscreen is so you need to make sure they have been absorbed.

Keeping the cost in mind when it comes to serums, if you're looking for one good all-rounder, I would always choose something with Vitamin A in it such as Environ AVST. I also like Neostrata serum or Pestle + Mortar Hyaluronic serum as good all-rounders. You want a serum that is lightening and gives clarity.

SPF

This is the last and most crucial step in your morning skincare routine. Sunscreen isn't a sexy skincare product. When I say sunscreen, people think of the white caste, the stickiness and thickness of it. They think

of their precious foundation sliding down into a pool at their ankles –
but you can stop thinking this. Contemporary sunscreens are *nothing*
like this, especially the ones intended for everyday use under makeup.
If you don't like the texture, you won't apply it regularly and brands know
that we are conscious of wearability, of consistency and of it causing
breakouts. The sunscreens that I recommend to people are essentially
just photoprotection fortified moisturisers with silky, dewy finishes or a
mattifying primer-type effect.

There are two forms of sunscreen: physical and chemical. You can get
sunscreens that are just physical or just chemical or a mixture of both. I
prefer to opt for a combination of physical and chemical together.

- **Physical**: Physical is the shield that sits on the top of the skin as
  though it is a layer of crushed mirrors bouncing the light back out into
  the atmosphere. They stop the rays from getting through to the skin.
- **Chemical**: Chemical sunscreen will absorb the rays from the sun and
  the body will then break it down and filter it through the body.

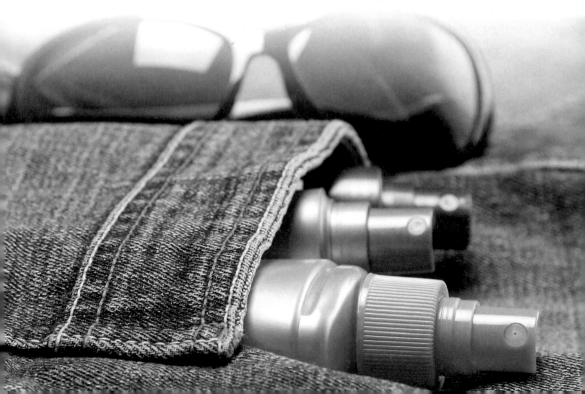

You won't really find a fully physical sunscreen apart from SkinCeuticals Mineral Radiance UV Defense, Avène Mineral Fluid SPF 50+ or Neostrata Sheer Physical Protection (by fully mineral, I mean all of the sun-blocking ingredients are mineral – these products do contain other chemicals for different purposes). Even sunscreens like my favourite IMAGE Prevention+ SPF 32 contain both physical and chemical blocks.

The reason I like the combination is so that I know I am fully covered.

If you went for purely physical, some rays may still get through as few of us apply enough sunscreen in every millimetre of skin where it's needed. For the rays that do seep through, the chemical part of the sunscreen will sort them out. It's a double whammy.

I opt for versions that are lightweight, moisturising, have filters and can sit under makeup. Ideally we should reapply throughout the day (every two hours) but this tends not to happen. Even if you're sitting indoors all day but you are staring at a computer screen, it's advised that you reapply so that you are protected from the HEV (High Energy Visible rays) given off by screens. Many brands now have sprays which are translucent so can be topped up without disturbing your makeup. There are also mineral SPF powders (Jane Iredale Powder Me SPF 30, Brush-On-Block SPF 30). These are translucent powders that offer light protection.

Purely chemical sunscreens are often the ones you find in supermarkets, they tend to be own-brand and cheaper. They're the ones you know from the telly, the ones you buy beside the beach. They need to be applied twenty minutes before you go out into the sun so that they have time to start working because they need to penetrate into the skin to protect from UV damage.

Application wise, you should be applying a teaspoon of sunscreen to your face, neck and ears – approximately half a teaspoon on your face alone. Don't massage it into your visage. When applying sunscreen, you're attempting to create a flawless protective shield across the skin so focus on getting every single square inch by smoothing it across the skin, a teaspoon per limb.

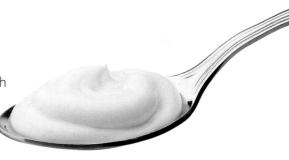

Many find this easiest to do with only two fingers. Go slow and steady and never ever mix it with another product as this can render it useless. It needs to be on you on its own as the final step prior to makeup application, if you apply makeup.

Don't forget to apply it on *all* areas that are exposed. Some days, this is just your face and hands if you are a Steve Jobs style turtleneck wearer. Other days, you'll have to include your shoulders. On the beach or in direct heated sunlight, it has to be *everywhere*.

Sunscreen isn't just to protect against skin cancer, which is a concern that should never be swept under the rug, it's also to protect you from light-related pigmentation, solar elastosis (aka the destruction of your elastin overtime leading to ridges, creases and a rubbery texture to the skin) and premature ageing in general.

You should be wearing sunscreen all day, every day. Full stop. I won't hear your 'buts'.

'But, Jenn, it's not sunny outside. Why do I need *sun* protection factor?'

It is not just sun protection factor, dear nerd, it is *light* protection factor. In countries like Ireland and the UK, we get UVB rays, the rays that cause skin cancer and sunburn, from April through to September. However, like everywhere else on the planet, we are hit by UVA rays all year round, through clouds and through windows, come rain, snow or shine. UVA rays can penetrate into the skin much deeper, all the way down into the dermis (see Skin Anatomy chapter) and damage it at a cellular level. UVA damage is what causes lax and crepe-like skin, pigmentation and a whole host of other photo-damage concerns. You need UVA protection all year round – even on Christmas Day – whereas UVB is only for the rays where you could burn ('A' is for ageing and 'B' is for burning).

UVA rays are the reason your everyday sunscreen needs to be broad spectrum. The factor system lets you know how well protected you are from UVB rays, but the UVA symbol (UVA with a circle around it) tells you that your sunscreen is truly broad spectrum and protects you from both. The other system is the star system, where a number of stars are awarded to an SPF going by the level of UVA protection compared to the level of UVB protection, with 5 being the best. An SPF of 50 with 5 stars has every high UVA protection, but an SPF of 15 with 5-star protection has much less UVA protection. Quiz the person selling the sunscreen to you to figure out the best option.

Chemical SPF ingredients, such as oxybenzone and octyl methoxycinnamate absorb UV rays and change them into low-level heat. These are known as organic because they contain carbon atoms which make up all organic matter – see the confusion when it comes to natural skincare?

Physical (mineral) SPF ingredients, such as zinc oxide and titanium dioxide, work to deflect UV rays from the skin and I would always look for these ingredients in my SPF

As a rule of thumb, I avoid an SPF that has a very long list of ingredients but is still heavy in antioxidants.

You'll often find both in an SPF to provide the best protection possible. Physical SPF protects you straight away, unlike chemical SPFs, which needs twenty minutes to start working, hence the benefits of including both in one product.

The Skin Nerd approved SPFs:

- Murad City Skin Age Defence Broad Spectrum SPF 50: This has UVA, UVB, HEV protection as well as antioxidants and a gorgeous texture.

- IMAGE Preventative+ Daily Matte Moisturiser SPF 32: This is good as it has microspheres that mop up excess oil; it's also good as a makeup primer.

- Avène Tinted Mineral Fluid SPF 50+: I like this because it's lightweight, cooling on the skin and you don't need to wear makeup with it.

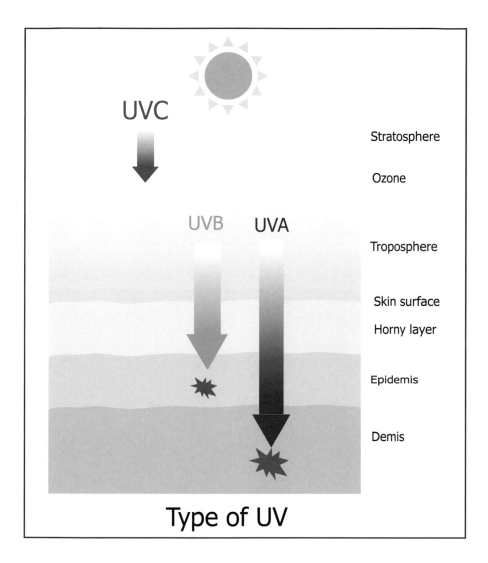

UVC

Stratosphere

Ozone

UVB UVA

Troposphere

Skin surface
Horny layer

Epidemis

Demis

Type of UV

UVA versus UVB

More UVA rays make it to the earth than UVB ones, so they pose a greater risk just because there are more of them. Because of their length, UVA rays can get deeper into your skin and cause age-related damage. Recently, it has been found that they are known to contribute to or cause all types of skin cancer too.

UVB rays are what come alongside heated sunlight of any kind, and are known to cause or contribute to skin cancer. They are what cause sunburn (and pigmentation). They are not the omnipresent risk that UVA rays are, but, like UVA rays, they can cause irreparable damage to the skin.

What about the SPF in your makeup?

Beauty brands love telling us that their products double as your primary SPF. Your foundation has SPF 30, you think. Well, nope, it doesn't.

For your SPF to work as your primary mode of light protection, you'd have to be wearing the suitable amount (as referenced earlier, a teaspoon for face, neck and ears). Nobody wears that much foundation evenly across their face. Nobody!

Also, even if your foundation has UVB protection, it probably doesn't have UVA protection. Sorry, not sorry.

Same goes for moisturiser. If it has a slightly tackier texture and you layer the recommended amount on to yourself, then, yes, it is a functional sunscreen. One of my all-time favourite sunscreens is marketed as a moisturiser (IMAGE Prevention SPF 32). However, you can tell by the mild stickiness before it dries in (seamlessly, may I add) that it is a true sunscreen.

Makeup is a nice additional layer to your sunscreen though, kind of like the goalie behind your defence on a football pitch. I do soccer-mom Saturdays with my aspiring mini Mo Salah, sincere apologies.

The ideal factor? You need to be using at least factor 30 but preferably factor 50 if you've ever reached for a foundation shade called 'porcelain', 'ivory' or 'alabaster'. Wearing factor 30 or factor 50 doesn't mean you get away with skimping on how much you use or that you don't have to reapply it.

UVA

And, to drive the point home, the key is less about the factor but more about using enough.

Has the SPF message sunk in? Good. Now we move on to add-ons.

Add-ons

Outside of the essentials mentioned above, there are skincare add-ons that you can opt for, depending on your skin concerns, such as exfoliation and the occasional overnight or sheet mask. Some of these are necessary, but they're not needed every morning and night.

Moisturiser

Shock horror. Moisturiser is not something I feel we need by day. Yet there are countless moisturisers on the market. In truth, we get everything we need from our serums and SPF, but, at night, when we don't need SPF, most of my clients will opt for a moisturiser purely because it feels delicious, soft, supple on their skin – and yet it does not serve a full purpose beyond that unless it mirrors the good fats, ceramides, in the skin.

I can understand why a low-in-lipids, dry-skinned people or an over-exfoliating individual would use a moisturiser as it provides instant comfort to the skin, but usually that all it does. The molecules in it are too big to penetrate the skin, which is why it can manage to stay in the upper layers and soften and condition them. You will notice a lot of SPFs now marketed as moisturisers as people want to buy moisturisers more than SPF: the IMAGE Prevention is a good example.

Exfoliator

Unfortunately, we have all been conditioned to over-exfoliate. We are obsessed with the need to exfoliate away our skin cells and feel that instant gratification of soft, supple, baby-soft skin. Companies teach us that for lighter, brighter and hydrated skin, exfoliation is the solution.

NO.

It is not. Short-term perhaps, but not long-term.

Certainly not to the extent we've been led to believe. The skin should be exfoliating itself, but because of lifestyle and chronological ageing, it tends to slow down from top to toe. We then lean on scrubs and grits to pummel the bejesus out of ourselves, stepping out of the shower all lobster like and congratulating ourselves on how clean we are – I call it raw. It's psychologically rewarding, but your skin won't thank you.

If you over-exfoliate, you deplete the natural oil levels that should be there. Oil is a friend to the skin, you may dislike it, but it is indeed a positive. With acne, if you over-exfoliate you may only further spread the bacteria. It is comparable to sandpapering and scouring an area that needs to be dissolved and the lumps and bumps can be removed from the inside out. Furthermore, with over-exfoliation, you also make the skin more prone to dehydration, to light sensitivity and oiliness (as your skin will just over-produce oil as a result). There is no positive to over-exfoliating.

How often should we exfoliate?

From the age of twenty-five, you should exfoliate no more than three times a week, leaving a night in between to enable your skin to rest!

Exfoliation isn't as necessary in those under twenty-five, as the skin's natural rate of exfoliation is doing A-OK, but, again, it depends on the individual's skin. Maybe once or twice a week is enough, or using an active cleanser alone would do the trick for most under twenty-five year olds. However, if your skin looks bright, not dull, and you don't have problems with acne or anything else, don't fret if you're not exfoliating.

When it comes to exfoliator types, I recommend a total ban on microbeads to save not just the fish but also your face. Microbeads are going to be banned in Ireland as fish and birds are eating them and it is causing them harm as they do not decompose in the digestive systems of the fishies and birds.

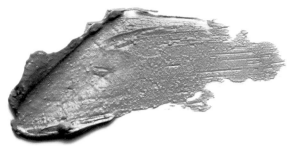

We don't need to use chunky gritty formulas to exfoliate properly. No exfoliating scrubs. Think of the top layer of your skin as tiles on a roof, then think of beads or grains constantly chipping away at the tile until eventually it cracks the grout. Bringing that analogy back to skin the grout being removed is comparable to the seal being broken and the protective layer being exposed. The skin then becomes dehydrated. Think of a glass of water left on a table, eventually the water will evaporate. The skin is comprised of water and so if the seal is left exposed that water too evaporates.

Your skin is acidic so applying a mild, skin-suited acid is okay. Much kinder than a scrub, in fact. The only exfoliators I recommend are acids or enzymes, or lightweight granules that don't remotely scratch the skin. Acids and enzymes don't chip off the tile, they drip through the cracks so they get in without causing damage and prompt the cells to slough off on their own from down below. In this sense, they are much more

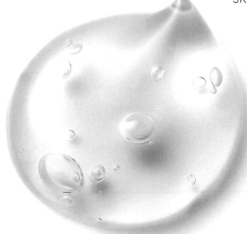

skin-friendly when used correctly. Examples of exfoliators I recommend include glycolic acid, lactic acid, polyhydroxy acids, salicylic acids and enzymatic exfoliation products that contain bromelain (pineapple enzyme) and papain (papaya enzyme) usually.

In terms of exfoliator rules, follow the box, bottle or packet. Exfoliators are all different and come in different formulations and percentages, so you really have to speak to the person who sold it to you. For the most part, it is best to use them post-cleansing and pre-seruming so that your pores are most receptive to the next products and they will penetrate deeper into the epidermis. It's best to exfoliate at night, which is what I do, so that you can then give your skin some respite while you sleep.

I believe acid-based exfoliators should only ever be retailed by those providing guidance. People will come to us saying they bought a peel solution online and it is clear that their skin's barrier has been compromised to the point of scaliness and flakiness all day, every day.

The Skin Nerd approved exfoliators:

- Murad Age Reform Hydro-Glow Aqua Peel
- Neostrata Glycolic Treatment Peel Kit
- Yon-Ka Gommage 305
- IMAGE Skincare Ageless Total Resurfacing Masque
- Ren Glycol Lactic Radiance Renewal Mask
- Environ Tri Biobotanical Revival Masque (formerly known as Intensive Revival Masque)

Masks

Masks are important to a skincare routine as they help us to get more actives onto our skin, and sometimes they perform a specific function as a boost to the skin that perhaps doesn't exist in your regular routine. Maybe your focus in your routine isn't hydration but one week you need a boost of hydration and this is where a mask may come in to play.

We don't need masks every day as we have daily skincare and it would be simply too much to include masks too (especially active masks). Natural masks could be used every day though, if you were so inclined. Realistically, I tell people to use them once or twice a week, depending on the type of mask (if active use it less, if inactive you could use it more often but there's no real need to do so).

It's important to be mindful of the fact that masks should be an add-on to a solid skincare routine. If you don't take care of your skin from one end of the week to the next and you slap on a mask hoping to make up for it, well that's just like leaving the house with a raincoat and no clothes on underneath. Masks are a quick fix but they are not long term. I might use a mask on a Thursday if I'm feeling tired and sluggish, and it's visible in my skin, and wake up on Friday morning looking rejuvenated.

Masks from a tub or a tube are probably the easiest product to apply. Apply a cherry-sized amount or a thick layer across the surface of your face and neck and leave it on for the time specified. Do not wear masks overnight unless it is clearly marked as an overnight mask or your therapist has advised you to do so.

An example of this would be the IMAGE Skincare Vital C Hydrating Overnight Masque or the Yon-Ka Masque No°1. These masks should be applied as above at the end of your normal night-time routine, but left on all night long, as Lionel Richie would say. You should cleanse the next day. I believe cleansing every morning is key, but your skin may be a tad oilier after using an overnight mask. Ensure you follow the instructions on the mask itself.

Sheet masks can be a bit fiddly. You need to take the mask out of its sachet carefully and give it a little swish around to collect the excess serum – here's a bonus tip, apply the serum that collects in the packet to arms, neck and legs before you apply the mask for maximum value.

Before applying your sheet mask, make sure you've peeled off anything that needs to be peeled off. Some sheet gel masks have a delicate plastic coating that has to be removed before it is used – I learned this the hard way.

Leave on the mask for the specified time. I usually go for thirty minutes dependent on the ingredients.

My top tip is to mask on planes, trains and automobiles. Because of the low-humidity cabin air and constantly-blasting air conditioning, planes suck moisture from the skin. I used to get off planes looking ten years older. A hydrating mask will combat this!

There are masks that target different concerns. Some claim to remove pores (and no that's not a typo, there are masks that suggest removing your pores entirely which just makes me laugh), while others are for illuminating or anti-ageing purposes (usually containing a blend of acids and antioxidants/peptides).

I strongly advise steering clear of charcoal masks that you pull off the face as they tend to take a lot more than just blackheads. They adhere to the skin too much and some of them contain a form of PVA glue. No thank you. The skin is an organ.

These are some of my favourite mask brands:

Sheet masks

- Seoulista Instant Facial Sheet Masks: These are good for brightening and luminosity.

- IMAGE I-MASK Biomolecular sheet masks: The quality and immediacy of results are brilliant.

- Primark/Penneys sheet masks: These are super-affordable and really do what they say.

- Charlotte Tilbury Revolutionary Instant Magic Facial Dry Sheet Masks: She has a dry mask which is good if you don't like all of that gloopiness.

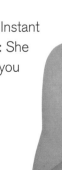

👓 THE SKIN NERD

I tend to opt for biocellulose sheet masks as they are made from natural materials – usually coconut shell – because these hold the lotion well.

Cream masks

- Environ Tri Biobotanical Revival Masque: This is brilliant for anti-ageing and works progressively. Leave it on for just ten minutes the first time you use it then increase over time until you can wear it throughout the night.

- Juliette Armand Elements Oxygen Foaming Mask: This is great for dewiness and freshness as it brings oxygen to the tissues.

- Rodial Vit C Brightening mask: This is good for brightening.

- IMAGE Clear Cell Clarifying Masque for acne prone skin: You can use this three ways: either mix it in with your Clear Cell cleanser to boost its efficacy, leave it on as a mask on its own for ten minutes before removing or dab it directly onto a spot.

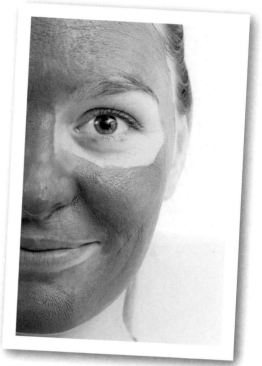

Clay masks

Most clay masks on the market are like vacuums and suck up far too much moisture, but if you fancy one, I recommend Yon-Ka as they offer a really good balance between clay and moisture. Remove by compressing or blotting moisture into the clay so it isn't scrubbed off, which leaves the skin visibly red.

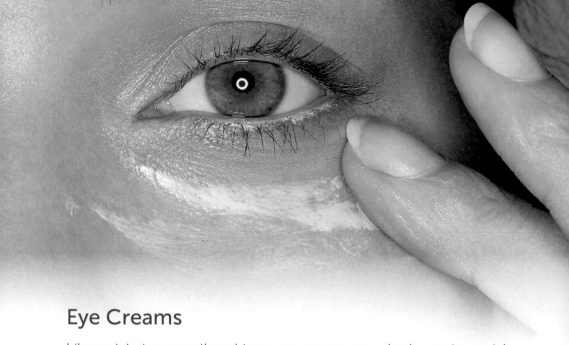

Eye Creams

Like moisturisers, my thoughts on eye creams may also be controversial. Essentially, eye creams contain the same, or similar, ingredients to the rest of your skincare, as they are usually built for the purpose of soothing puffiness, reducing the appearance of lines or to tackle dark circles (i.e. increase blood flow to the skin, as topical caffeine does).

The pain is that many eye creams say that you can't use them close to the eye – hello? Am I missing something here? It is an eye cream, not a cheekbone cream. My cheekbone doesn't have dark circles.

I don't believe that eye creams are essential if you're using good serums. They can double as your eye cream as long as it says they can be used up close to the eye. Eye creams are usually heavy in peptides (collagen stimulating amino acids on a mission – they are a bossy-boot cell that wants their job done), which you are getting in most anti-ageing products anyway, as well as general hydrating ingredients, like hyaluronic acid, and vitamins, such as A, C and E, which are also probably in your routine. Personally, I don't see enough of a difference with most eye creams to justify them, and I have a natural indent just under my eyes so I am a prime candidate.

That said, if you're an eye-cream fiend, one eye cream that I've always found effective is the Environ Vita-Peptide Eye Gel. It contains three patented peptides – Matrixyl® 3000, Argireline® and Dermaxyl® – which stimulate the production of collagen and elastin, reduce the contraction of muscles to slow the formation of lines and wrinkles and help the skin to make ceramides to keep the skin plump. It also contains Vitamins A, C and E for their normalising and antioxidant properties. Yes, it is the exact ingredient that I previously listed as pointless in an eye cream but you don't find such a potent blend of peptides often and I've used it and seen the results so I will vouch for it. It also has botox-mimicking properties.

I also like Pestle + Mortar Renew which contains caffeine. Caffeine applied topically is great for dark circles. I also like Yon-Ka Nutri Contour as it is extremely hydrating, good for dryness or irritated eyes. It's very comforting on the eye area. And, for a general quick fix, I like IMAGE Illuma eye cream. If you don't feel the need for this additional step don't worry, you should be getting what you need from your serum.

Spot Treatments

When many hear 'spot treatment', they presume it is just for literal spots as in pimples. But this is not necessarily the case. There are also spot treatments for pigmentation and many will spot-apply treatments for localised redness. Use spot treatments sparingly, especially when it comes to acid or peptide-based ones. They are usually mega concentrated so you only need a tiny drop, probably smaller than you think. Dab it on or give it a rub in if the instructions say to. This will usually slot into your daily routine, morning and evening, or just evening, depending on the specific product itself.

When it comes to acne treatments, you can hold them to the spot with your finger, cotton pad or cotton swab for a few seconds. Do not pre-emptively cover your face in acne spot treatments as it may just dry out and aggravate your skin; only use them directly on spots and blackheads. You can apply your acne spot treatment morning and night or if you have a particularly nasty one to get rid of, you can reapply it throughout the day. Take my warning though: spot treatments will cause dryness if used too often.

Spritz O'Clock

Spritz O'Clock is the Nerdie name for using a facial mist. My favourite day time treat. There are two types of spritzes: hydrating and medicinal.

Hydrating spritzes are those that provide purely hydration and little else. The best example would be Avène's Eau Thermale spring water. This not only hydrates the skin but contains anti-inflammatory microflora which limits itching and irritation.

Medicinal spritzes can actively improve the skin rather than solely hydrating it. Sometimes, they contain blends of essential oils for healing and soothing properties, such as my personal favourite Lotion Yon-Ka and, sometimes, they are pollution-protectants or for barrier repair, such as Dermalogica's UltraCalming Mist.

Spritzing can help to bring additional hydration to your skin throughout the day, set makeup and 'wake up' makeup after you've been wearing it for a few hours. You can spritz as often as possible – I keep one in the car, one in my handbag and about three on my desk. There's no such thing as too many Spritz O'Clocks.

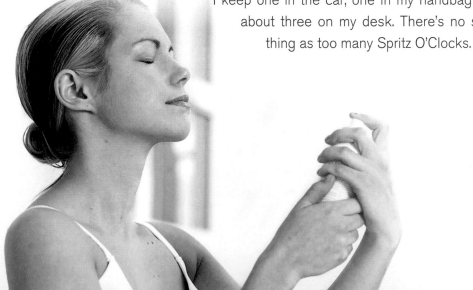

The Skin Nerd approved brands

Across the board, whether you're looking for a cleanser or a serum or a spritz o'clock product, these are the existing brands that I highly recommend:

- Murad
- IMAGE Skincare
- Environ
- SkinCeuticals
- Académie Scientifique de Beauté
- Yon-Ka
- Neostrata
- Marie Reynolds (Dermabiome)
- Drunk Elephant
- Medik8
- Danné Montague King
- Alpha - H
- No 7
- Avène

Can I use more than one brand?

Yes, because the ingredients are more important than the brand. Some people say they have 'tried it all', or that they cleanse, tone and moisturise, but the reason they have purchased these products is often only because they trust a luxury brand, and not the powerhouse ingredients inside.

Makeup

Many people see skincare as an addition to makeup or a quick thing to prepare the skin for makeup application. However, beauty professionals, like facialists, dermatologists and aestheticians, have, for years, decried makeup as something that can only detract from your skincare and promoting going makeup-free as something to aspire to.

It is certainly a tricky topic but, in the end, it comes down to the type of makeup you are using. I am a huge advocate for mineral makeup as it gives back to the skin in a way that cosmetic makeup truly cannot. When you're using the right type of makeup, it acts as a barrier to protect the skin from dust, pollution and the rigors of everyday life. It can also act as a backup dancer to the Britney Spears that is your everyday sunscreen.

Most of us wear makeup for ten or so hours a day – pretty much our entire waking existence. Think about that if you don't think the makeup you're using matters.

The best makeup for your skin is fully mineral makeup, but, first, we need to discuss cosmetic makeup for a second.

Cosmetic makeup

Cosmetic makeup is makeup created by large house brands. It makes up the majority of what you find in department stores, chemists and shops.

Cosmetic makeup – unlike its angelic counterpart, mineral makeup – sits in the pore. In itself, cosmetic makeup isn't harmful for the skin but it doesn't provide benefits for it either. I personally find cosmetic makeup to be quite drying because of the high levels of drying alcohols, like denatured alcohol, pigment with no added purpose and sensitising fragrances they contain.

Cosmetic makeup is also heavy in talc. Now, talc is technically a mineral but it is a mineral that does little bar dry out the skin. It is added to products to help them to give the skin a matt look or to bulk out the product (as it's a highly affordable ingredient). So a product can say that they are mineral but most of that mineral could be talc, so you need to be wary of that too.

Watch out for ingredients marked as 'parfum', fragrance or perfume, denatured alcohol/alcohol denat /SD alcohol and silicones. As you know from your reading, this type of alcohol and fragrances can dehydrate the skin and damage its barrier, leading to all sorts of skin hassle. Silicones are known to be quite comedogenic (aka pore-clogging) so are best to be avoided.

All in all, fragrances, alcohol and other ingredients that dry out and sensitise the skin can also speed up the skin's ageing process, which actually begins around twenty-five. The youths think that they can get away with

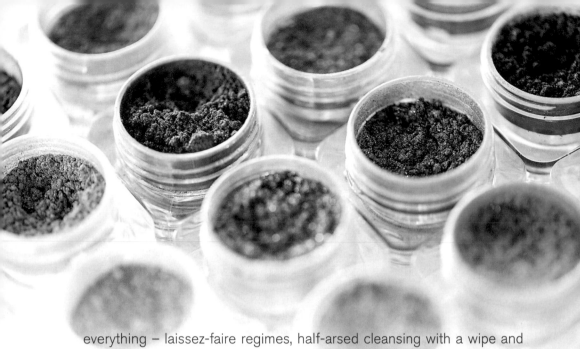

everything – laissez-faire regimes, half-arsed cleansing with a wipe and caking on the cosmetic makeup – but, perhaps, their skin is not as youthful as they think!

The fact that mineral makeup is preferable is no secret. Even the large house brands have realised this and have started marketing to that effect with 'mineralised' products. Some brands market their products as mineral brands even though their products are not fully mineral. There is, unfortunately, no regulation on how much mineral a product must contain for it to be able to be labelled as such. Mineralised products are simply cosmetic products with added minerals.

In my eyes, it is like placing one diamond into a predominantly cubic zirconia tiara and then selling it as a 100 per cent real diamond tiara. The consumer usually has no notion of how little mineral is actually in the product.

Mineral makeup – and by mineral I mean wholly mineral – is beneficial for the skin in a number of ways. Minerals like zinc oxide and titanium oxide, which are also found in sunscreen, are naturally photo-protective and antioxidant in nature. Minerals hydrate the skin and can also mattify it. Minerals sit on the pore rather than in the pore because of their larger molecular size and so do not cause congestion or interrupt the skin's natural processes of secretion and protection. In this sense, they work with the skin rather than against it.

I fully understand why many are put off mineral makeup before they have even seen it. Marketing has led us to believe that it is for more mature skin and that it is only available in low-coverage powder formulations. You should cut out that thinking *now*. Some brands, such as Jane Iredale, have full ranges of mineral products with multiple liquid and powder foundations, blushes, lipsticks, eyeliners, contour kits, highlighters and primers.

Mineral powders are not like setting powders. They're a different breed altogether and are truly buildable. You can pop one layer on for a general sheath of coverage or you can layer it up good for a night out. If you are spot-prone, mineral powders are fabulous for spot concealing as you can use a delicate brush with a small head to build cover seamlessly in one specific area. As minerals are naturally anti-inflammatory, mineral makeup will actually help the spot itself. It's what dreams are made of.

If you really cannot be swayed to a powder, there are also beautifully full coverage matte and hydrating mineral liquid foundations out there.

Using 'bad' makeup with a good skincare routine is a counterproductive. Why put time, money and effort into trying to stay young looking and clearing out your pores only to contribute to your skin's ageing process and spackle up your pores?

My favourite mineral brands would be Jane Iredale, with whom I worked with very closely for years, and Bellapierre, whom I also love. They aren't the same as many famed mineral brands, but they use high-quality minerals and work on creating the best formulations they can.

There is no harm in having completely makeup-free days but if you are wearing mineral makeup, it doesn't really matter. In fact, wearing this make-up can act as a barrier. I do feel like being makeup-free is good for the soul though. If you only wear cosmetic makeup, take it off as early in the evening as you can. Or if you have a day at home, try and give it a break. The more your skin improves as you follow the advice in this book, the less scary the make-up free idea will be. I promise.

My makeup routine

After my skincare routine, which finishes with an SPF, I move onto makeup.

My personal favourite primer (though not sold as a primer) is IMAGE Prevention+ Daily Matte Moisturiser SPF 32. It provides a nice velvety matte base for makeup to adhere to properly and keeps my makeup where I want it all day long.

Your sunscreen should always be your last step before your makeup, unless you use a spray sunscreen that can be used on top of makeup. Jane Iredale and Bellapierre both have mineral primers too for both dewy or matte finishes.

When it comes to eye makeup, I use regular cosmetic makeup – this is certainly not my strong point. I finish off the look with a mineral blush and spritz with my Spritz O'Clock (your preferred facial mist, NOT setting spray – alcohol ahoy!) to set it and add a bit more topical hydration.

To remove makeup, my preferred mode is the Cleanse Off Mitt®, although I am biased. I first wet my mitt, wring it out and then pop it on my hand. Then I gently swipe it across my skin first to remove my foundation and blush and things like that. When that's done, I flip the COM over and take off my eye makeup gently with the clean side by rolling it downwards over my lashes gently so as not to damage them. I follow this up with my traditional cleanser and rinse 'til all residue is gone – ta-da!

Dirty makeup brushes are a lovely, easy way to introduce lots of bacteria to your skin, the worst-case scenario being ending up with a staph infection on your face. Yikes. This is why the pros are always telling you to clean them. They aren't just trying to make your life miserable – the added bonus is that clean makeup brushes apply makeup better!

I personally use a daily brush cleansing spray, such as Ella & Jo Squeaky Clean Brush Cleanser and then wipe them over clean tissue paper or kitchen roll (sometimes, out of use Cleanse Off Mitts®). All that really matters is that what you're using to clean your makeup brushes is antibacterial (sorry, baby shampoo lovers).

Why is it so important? Well, we are often not so hygienic with our makeup brushes – plenty of people have them out in the open in their bathroom or at the bottom of dirty handbags (no judgement on the handbag dirt though, we all have dirty handbags).

Sample Skincare Routines

Lucy's Weekly Routine

Lucy is twenty-three, so her own production of collagen and elastin hasn't slowed down yet – jealous, much? She suffers from congestion and as she says herself, it is hormone related. Her main goals for her skin are to prevent spots from forming and help to clear up her post-inflammatory hyperpigmentation.

Lucy is very, very pale and quite prone to pigment forming so she is willing to spend time on her routine. She has reluctantly switched to mineral makeup and has found that it CAN give full coverage and have a nice finish.

An hour after putting on her makeup, she will have a bit of oil accumulating around her nose and on her forehead and by the end of the day, she's lucky if there is any part of her face left matte. The vast majority of her congestion would be found on the lower half of her face, usually on her jawline but also on her chin, around the mouth and sometimes under her cheekbones. In hot weather, she finds that she'll break out on her forehead and between her eyebrows.

Monday to Sunday	
Morning	• Environ B-Active Sebuwash Cleansing Gel (mild, tea tree and salicylic): cleanser to clear out the pore of debris and regulate oil
	• Waxperts Wonder Pads (salicylic acid spot treatment): to apply directly to spots as an extra boost of salicylic acid, to dry them out and bring them down
	• Environ SkinEssentiA Vita-Antioxidant AVST Moisturiser 1 (vitamin A serum): for general skin health and repair on a cellular level
	• Environ Vita-Enriched Colostrum gel: to introduce growth factors for better skin healing mixed with IMAGE Ageless Hyaluronic Filler (hyaluronic serum) for hydration and plumpness
	• Murad City Skin Broad Spectrum SPF 50 for broad spectrum protection from UV and HEV (blue light)
	• Jane Iredale Glow Time BB Cream foundation step 1
	• Jane Iredale PurePressed Powder foundation step 2

Monday to Sunday	
Evening	• Pre-cleanse with Cleanse Off Mitt®
	• Environ B-Active Sebuwash Cleansing Gel
	• Waxperts Wonder Pads
	• Environ SkinEssentiA Vita-Antioxidant AVST Moisturiser
	• Environ Vita-Enriched Colostrum gel mixed with IMAGE Ageless Hyaluronic Filler (hyaluronic serum) for hydration and plumpness

Add-ons/Changes

Monday & Tuesday evening: At the end of her routine on these evenings, Lucy applies the Yon-Ka Masque No° 1 (to sleep in) for a quick mega boost of hydration. If over-used it would trigger breakouts.

Tuesday & Saturday evening: Lucy switches from the Sebuwash Clearing Gell to the IMAGE Clear Cell Cleanser on these evenings — this is , a strong, highly active salicylic cleanser for exfoliation and a stronger clearing power. This product is too strong to use every day so she sticks with twice a week with a break of three days in between.

Thursday & Sunday evening: Following her cleanse, Lucy uses the Neostrata Glycolic Daily Peel Pad (exfoliator) for additional exfoliation only on areas of scarring, to improve cell turnover and help to bring pigment up through the layers of the skin. If over-used, it would cause congestion.

Friday evening: Lucy applies the Seoulista Instant Facial Super Hyaluronic Sheet Mask (hydrating sheet mask) at the end of her routine for a pre-going out burst of hydration so that makeup sits better and skin looks its best in a jiffy.

*Supplements wise, Lucy also takes 2 x Skin Accumax in the AM with breakfast and 2 with dinner, 7 days a week.

Paula's Weekly Routine

Paula is 46 years of age and as most people in their forties who haven't religiously worn sunscreen since birth, she has sun damage and hyper-pigmentation in the form of small dark spots across her face. She has some lines and wrinkles around her eyes, on her forehead and around her mouth.

When she was younger, she used to suffer from oily skin so she's fond of a wash-type cleanser but prior to this routine, she was using products that dehydrated her skin so it felt tight after washing it and looked dull. She lives in the city centre and walks through the city for work five days a week, so she is exposed to your typical city pollutants.

Monday to Sunday	
Morning	• X1 Skinade Collagen Drink shot – to boost collagen production and skin hydration from the inside
	• X 1 Advanced Nutrition Programme Skin Vit A + – for internal vitamin A
	• Murad Essential C Cleanser – a gentle wash that doesn't dehydrate the skin and contains antioxidants A, C & E to tackle free radical damage

	## Monday to Sunday
	• SkinCeuticals CE Ferulic – highly potent vitamin C/ antioxidant serum that improves pigmentation and also battles free radicals • Environ Skin EssentiA Vita-Antioxidant AVST Moisturiser 5 • Murad City Skin SPF 50+ – broad spectrum SPF that also protects from blue light/HEV
Evening	• Pre-cleanse with Cleanse Off Mitt® • Murad Essential C Cleanser – a gentle wash that doesn't dehydrate the skin and contains antioxidants A, C & E to tackle free radical damage • Neostrata Enlighten Illuminating Serum – tyrosinase inhibitor aka stops the enzyme that creates pigment from working, brightening serum • Environ Skin EssentiA Vita-Antioxidant AVST Moisturiser 5 • Murad Hydro-Dynamic Ultimate Moisture – hyaluronic acid moisturiser to bring up epidermal hydration and support skin's barrier
Just Monday & Friday	Image Ageless Total Facial Cleanser – glycolic acid cleanser for exfoliation
When Needed	MooGoo SPF 15 Lip Balm – mineral filter sunscreen for lips

Charlotte's Weekly Routine

Charlotte is 32 years of age with naturally gorgeous skin. She's a very normal skin type (though we don't believe in skin type alone, remember?) that sometimes veers to dryness and her skin is a bit sensitive so that causes some redness and heat in her cheeks. She is line-free, the clarity of her skin is great with little to no pigmentation and she has a glow to her skin, perhaps due to her plant-based diet. She doesn't really wear makeup except for special events.

In skin like this, we are predominantly trying to protect it from damage and balance out any minor problems, such as Charlotte's reactivity. However, another thing to note is that Charlotte gets home from work late and doesn't want a long, long routine so this is quite basic to ensure that she doesn't have to do a whole lot.

Monday to Sunday	
Morning	<ul><li>IMAGE Vital C Hydrating Facial Cleanser – Vitamin C cleanser for antioxidant protection, hydration and to bring down any redness</li><li>Environ Skin EssentiA AVST Moisturiser 2 – Charlotte has moved on to the second step of the AVST series, Vitamin A is key for all skin</li><li>Skin Vit A x1 after eating, Skin Omegas x1 after eating</li></ul>

Monday to Sunday	
Evening	• Skin Omegas x1 after eating
	• Pre-cleanse with Cleanse Off Mitt® – to remove traces of pollution and grime from the face
	• IMAGE Vital C Hydrating Facial Cleanser – Vitamin C cleanser for antioxidant protection, hydration and to bring down any redness
	• Environ Skin EssentiA AVST Moisturiser 2 – Charlotte has moved on to the second step of the AVST series, Vitamin A is key for all skin
Saturday Evening	• Seoulista Super Hydration Instant Facial – hyaluronic acid sheet mask for a quick boost of hydration and a plump up

Charlotte home-rolls her AVST in on Monday and Thursday with the Environ Cosmetic Roll – CIT®. Hypothetically, Charlotte could be using a few other products if she was up for it. She could add in IMAGE Ormedic Balancing Antioxidant Serum for additional antioxidant protection and for its soothing qualities or an exfoliating product but that's not her style and that's okay. We have to make the regime affordable, accessible and realistic.

*These products were chosen following a detailed Nerdie consult and are for reference only.

Your Daily Checklist

Morning	• Cleanse • Serum & spot treatments • SPF • (Mineral makeup, optional) • Take your supplements as advised
Evening	• Take your supplements as advised • Pre-cleanse • Cleanse • Serum & spot treatments • Overnight mask/moisturiser, as required

Anti-Ageing Skincare

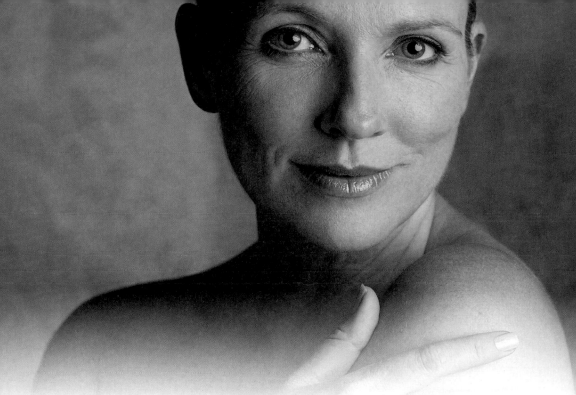

Everything you've read thus far contributes towards youthful healthy skin but for those who are mostly concerned with skin ageing, this chapter will give a quick overview of what you can do.

Ageing is literally a fact of life. As humans, we age. Fact. We can't stop this, we've no way to do that … that I know of. PS. If anyone does know, please contact me by whatever means necessary. Our skin ages too. Ageing has been vilified in popular media. You open up a magazine, or more realistically, you read an online article entitled 'Ex-Supermodel's Guide To Porcelain, Tight, Plump, Line-Free, Spot-Free, Plastic-Looking Skin' or 'Jesus, Isn't SHE Looking Haggard Now?'. How are you supposed to feel as a real human being who doesn't have literal millions to halt the ageing process?

Growing old gracefully is a positive thing, a gift. The accumulated smile lines and frown lines show everything you've been through in your life, mapping out the trials, tribulations and triumphs that you've come across. The problem is in accelerated ageing – we're cool with getting lines when we're supposed to but why let that happen if we can easily protect ourselves by making lifestyle changes and using antioxidants?

If you want to look your age, you can't be neglecting all that protecting.

The Ageing Process

Now, we don't have exact times for when the skin begins to age in different ways as everyone is different, so times given are estimates. Just take it that after 25, your skin slows down on carrying out the functions that keep it looking as good as it did before. Nice one, skin.

25 years of age: You have stopped creating collagen. Have a party but then quickly start taking Vitamin C supplements or collagen supplements and blast yourself with antioxidants daily to stop the collagen you have left from degrading. This is when you need to add the protection elements to your skincare, such as the aforementioned antioxidants (the ingredients usually considered to be anti-ageing). Even though you're probably not thinking about ageing right now, it's a myth that you don't need to worry about the ageing of your skin just yet. Start using Vitamin A serum now – it's never too early. Prevention of wrinkles and fine lines is key, and you can use it forever anyway.

30 years of age: Your skin's process of proliferation is slowing down. You're making fewer skin cells and getting rid of them slower. Your skin's collagen and elastin has decreased. You are now seeing fine lines around areas of expression like the forehead, maybe around the lips and around the eyes. At this point, you should perhaps be taking exfoliation more seriously, if you don't already, as your skin needs a bit of a hand in this area. However, this does not mean over-exfoliating! Additionally, hyaluronic acid and peptides will help to blur out those lines.

40 years of age: The rate at which your collagen is degrading increases rapidly. This is where your skin will start to look less plump, with hollows and creases like the nasolabial crease (leading from your nostril to the side of your mouth) will become more pronounced. Your skin may start to sag around the jawline. If you didn't bring those peptides in your 30s, now is the time to start and the same goes for hyaluronic acid. Your lymphatic system is slowing down too so pay attention to the sections on body brushing and facial massage to learn about how to kickstart it.

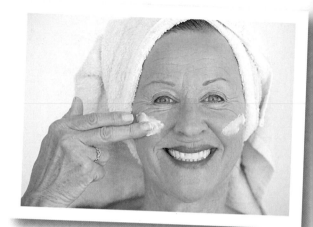

60 years of age: No more oestrogen! Because of this, your skin will be dryer than before. For some, this may mean switching to creamier, more hydrating cleansers, introducing more hyaluronic acid, and adding in moisturisers that can give you more lipids (which you lose some of when your oestrogen levels drop). Your lipids are the skin's good fats and they are essential for protecting it and stopping it from losing any more moisture.

When Should Anti-Ageing Efforts Begin?

Twenty-five is the age to consider starting your anti-ageing efforts, as that is the age when the proteins in your skin start to diminish. Deciphering whether or not you are dealing with accelerated ageing or chronological ageing (which is the usual rate of ageing and how we should age as per our genetics) can only be monitored by aesthetics. Have you significant redness? A prolonged tan? Open pores? A drop in elasticity beyond your years? If you had to look at your friends at a similar age (which is something we all do) how do you compare? Are you the harsh party life-styler, the neglected skin soul, the youthful one or the just-about-your-age look?

Best Treatments Specifically For Anti-Ageing

LED treatment
The red light in LED treatment can stimulate the fibroblast cell, the cell that makes up a huge part of the connective tissue of the skin and produces collagen. This makes it perfect for improving the tone and texture of ageing skin.

Ultherapy
Excellent for collagen boosting and reducing the appearance of sagging skin.

Microneedling
As microneedling also triggers the cascade of collagen, it's another great anti-ageing treatment.

Electrical muscle stimulation
This is fabulous for helping with facial structure as it targets the muscles under the skin itself.

Best Skingredients Specifically For Anti-Ageing

Peptides are an anti-ageing game changer so long as they are peptides that actually do something. When it comes to anti-ageing peptides, you're looking for peptides that send messages to your skin telling it to create collagen, as that is the key thing you're losing as you age.

Antioxidants of any and all kinds are required to defend against accelerated ageing (see p.44-47). As they protect the skin from free radical damage, they stop our collagen and elastin from degrading too soon, giving us more time with them.

Hyaluronic acid is often touted as anti-ageing skincare as we make less of it ourselves as we age. It also instantaneously plumps up the skin and keeps the skin feeling and looking supple, providing a short-term moisture gain.

Vitamin A is of course one of the best-known anti-ageing ingredients (see 'Vitamin A') and probably my number one, 'if you're not going to use anything else' recommendation for anti-ageing (after sunscreen, duh).

On that note, sunscreen. UV rays attack the things that make our skin look young so wearing sunscreen religiously from a young age is more than necessary, in my opinion.

Botox

Botox is the quickest of fixes to get rid of fine lines or wrinkles – I won't deny that. However, it's not a long-term solution. Botox is a neurotoxin known as botulinum toxin. When injected into the muscles underlying the skin, it stops them from receiving signals to move. When these muscles can't move, the wrinkles already there will fade and more wrinkles can't form in the area too. You're still able to feel in the area - it's a different type of nerve that is paralysed.

Everyone has their own opinion and can do as they will but what irks me about it is that it doesn't actually fix

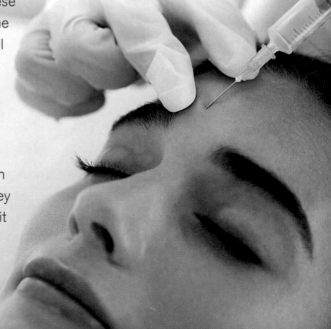

or prevent something if it isn't in your system. The effects of injections last about three to four months so you need to have it done again repeatedly.

I have tried it and the first time, holy moly, I was not me! I looked distorted. I tried it as I believe that for me to understand something properly, I need to walk the walk. **Disclaimer:** I don't try things if they are a) illegal or b) damaging to my health. There are practitioners out there who opt for what they dub as 'baby botox', which is a more natural, non-frozen look.

If you are looking into botox, opt for a cosmetic doctor who will be able to visualise how botox will affect your specific face rather than a doctor who will look at your face and say 'logically, we should put botox in point X and Y'.

As botox paralyses the muscle, the fear that I have is that it actually doesn't make the skin itself look younger. A great place to witness this is the Tube in London (people-watching is a hobby) – you see many people with facial muscles that seem to be ten years younger than their skin itself, yet the skin on top is coarse and needs TLC. People think that botox is an anti-ageing skin treatment but actually it's a stand-alone solution that doesn't address skin concerns. It can be used in tandem with products and treatments that are building up the health of your skin.

Our face ages on three levels: muscular, tissue and lymphatically. Within this there are texture, colouration and secretions. Some skin will get rougher, coarser and thicker, some will become pigmented or vascular (red, seeing broken capillaries), and some will make more or less oil. Getting botox is just targeting the muscle, skincare will target the tissue so long as it is bespoke and active and then jade stone and lymphasising are key for the lymphatic system. If you know about lymphasising, I am fairly impressed. Lymphasising means kickstarting the lymphatic system as it doesn't have a pump so you gotta do it yourself manually, hence why I do manual facial massage in the morning. You lymphasise by doing something called rebounding which is literally jumping up and down on a little trampoline. Bouncing against the surface of something gets the lymphatic system going, helping to relieve puffiness and detox us, carrying lymph towards the heart.

Targeting one of these facets alone is not enough – you need to work on them in synergy with each other for the best results.

Botox Versus Fillers

Getting dermal fillers means injecting hyaluronic acid or other ingredients, using their plumping abilities to plump to the maximum within the skin. Dermal fillers are used to restore volume rather than paralyse anything. Often, it'll be injected into wrinkles and lines to fill them out but it can also be used to subtly change the shape of your nose, for example, or to fill under-eye hollows (tear troughs) to reduce the appearance of dark circles in those who have a genetic indent. Perhaps fillers are most commonly known for the effect that they can have in largening the lips.

The effects of fillers last between a year and a half to two years, depending on where you're having filled in. Once again, like botox, fillers aren't treating the causes of the problem. They are not introducing collagen to your skin.

Rather than turning to botox or fillers alone as your first port of call, I advise first trying home EMS devices, such as Nu Face, which will exercise the muscles in the face using electric impulses and facial yoga.

I believe products and treatments are advanced enough now that we shouldn't need botox alone – though, it is needed in some cases if the client is particularly conscious and feels the need to change the muscle reaction dramatically. The frozen look is outdated and often not human-like in appearance.

However, if you are considering botox or fillers, make sure you seek a professional consultation with an expert.

We hear a lot about the importance of 'ageing gracefully', but I think this should be all about your state of mind. Feeling confident and good about your appearance and, more importantly, your skin health is what really matters.

Skin Conditions

Skin conditions can be something that happens once, rarely, or persistently and chronically throughout someone's life. You may get a rash once and never again. On the other hand, you may have psoriasis, an autoimmune disease, which must be managed on an ongoing basis. Skin concerns – rather than skin conditions – is an umbrella term that includes both more severe conditions but also more aesthetic quibbles, such as fine lines or laxity of the skin. It is all skin health though, make no mistake.

The number one thing that people don't do when they have a skin condition is to look for proper treatment. If you think you have rosacea, moderate to severe acne, psoriasis, melasma or eczema, you should visit your GP. As will be discussed repeatedly and at length in this book, everything is connected and the source of the condition is rarely the skin itself.

I have so many clients who come to me and say, 'I have rosacea' and, when I ask them about their diagnosis, more often than not, they tell me that they've never been formally diagnosed. Red cheeks does not rosacea make – you need a formal diagnosis.

Self-diagnosis is a true skin sin.

If you're having ongoing skin issues that you haven't been able to resolve, or you think you may have an issue that will require extra help, it's always a good idea to book yourself in for a consultation. Depending on the issue, we (The Skin Nerd team) can tell you whether or not you need to see a GP or a dermatologist. Ultimately, this book is a complementary guide to what we always advise at The Skin Nerd: a one-to-one consultation. In my Nerdie opinion, a thorough skin consultation with a licensed professional is the true key to skin health. If I could analyse each and every reader's exact skin through this book, I would. But it's personal.

When it comes to recommending specific products and treatments for people, many factors need to be considered. So think of this book as a fabulous starting point, and if you're serious about your skin, consider a consultation too.

Scarring

When you first get a wound, you need to treat it with care. It's an injury, it's an opening in the protective shield that is your skin, and you need to ensure that no more trauma befalls it so that it can heal as well as possible. Restrict movement as much as you can in the area and cover it when you're showering, if possible, because shower gels can irritate wounds – a plastic bag and a rubber band could do the trick. Keep it out of the sun as scars are much more sensitive to light.

Scarring is the skin's natural wound repair. It is dependent on:

- **Ethnicity**: Darker skin tones are more prone to losing pigment in the wound area and, as a result, it appears white, which means there is no protection in this area at all.
- **The depth of the wound**: The deeper and longer it is, the more inflammation has occurred and the more likely you'll be left with a scar.
- **Location of the wound**: If a wound is in a sun-exposed area, it is more likely to have PIH (post-inflammatory pigmentation), which is marking left after inflammation has occurred.
- **Genetics**: Healing ability can be dictated by the traits we've inherited. Blame your folks!
- **Diet**: Yes, what you eat can impact on scarring. A diet of processed food won't lend itself kindly to the knotting together and rehabilitation of the skin cell. Oops!
- **Infection**: If a wound becomes infected the probability of scarring is higher because the inflammation has increased and spread beyond the wound.

There are different type of scarring:
- acne pocks (indented)

- hypertrophic (a surgery scar)
- hair-removal scars (if the laser was too strong or the skin was not prepared correctly)
- stretch marks
- keloid, the overgrowth of tissue beyond the wound that leaves the scarred part of skin looking raised and puffy.

In terms of products, there isn't evidence that Vitamin E treatments or oils work for scarring, but many people find results with it, specifically when it comes to scars that are only healing or early stretch marks. This is when the scars are still pinkish, purplish or red rather than silver or white. Scarring, especially textural scarring like keloid scars, is caused by collagen that has formed too quickly in the healing process. As such, a lot more can be done in a salon or clinic than can be done at home. You may be able to get steroid injections from your GP or dermatologist, and laser therapy can also help as it targets the blood vessels in the scar tissue. There's also cryotherapy (freezing the scar), micro needling which stimulates the growth of collagen and elastin in the dermis, and surgical options, where people have dermal fillers for pitted scars.

Telangiectasia

This is the incredibly nerdie word for broken capillaries, which look like tiny red/purple lines across the skin, sometimes like webbing moving outwards from the original site. The capillaries tend to collapse or break because of pressure, friction and, in my opinion, a deficiency of Vitamin C.

Telangiectasia is also known as 'spider veins' because they can resemble a spider's web, and are like a milder form of varicose veins. Varicose veins, which are a dark-purple colour, are more common in people who are overweight. Spider veins are smaller and closer to the surface of the skin and are usually red or blue. They also look like tree

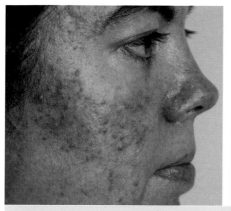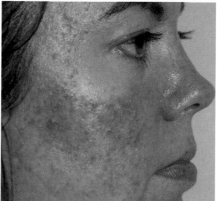

This client has suffered chronically with redness (rather than rosacea) and although the second image may seem like a marginal difference, it is definitely an improvement via a simple yet effective regimen over eight weeks. It is one step closer to life-changing.

branches and can cover either a small or large surface area. Spider veins affect most people, usually around the feet, legs and hips but you'd have to be up close to see them. You will often see spider veins wherever there has been a trauma to the skin. Spider veins can also be caused by sun exposure, especially on the face.

When it comes to prevention of varicose veins and spider veins, you need to focus on attempting to strengthen the veins and deal with any inflammation.

To do this, you need to provide your body with the following:

- **Bioflavonoids/flavonoids**: Bioflavonoids are compounds with antioxidant, anti-inflammatory and anti-viral properties that help to take strain from the blood vessels, aid in circulation and reduce blood pressure in the arteries. You can get your helping through root vegetables, such as carrots and turnips, soybeans, tea, broccoli, aubergine and flax seeds.
- **Vitamin C:** Vitamin C strengthens veins and fights inflammation and

you can get it from peppers, kale, broccoli, papaya, strawberries and Brussels sprouts to name but a few – however, I would not recommend eating them all together!

- **Regular exercise**: Exercising helps to get that blood pumping through your veins, which aids with strengthening.
- **Compression stockings**: They may not be the most attractive but slapping them on when you can (i.e. in the comfort of your own home) is key to preventing the formation of varicose veins and spider veins.

Salon treatment options for spider veins include:
- **EVLT (Endovenous Laser Ablation) with Nd:YAG laser**: The Nd-YAG laser involves a catheter being guided into the affected areas. A tiny laser is passed through the catheter and seeks out the colour of the blood in the vein. Then, bursts of energy heat and seal the vein. The blood and fragments of vein are later removed by the body's scavenger cells. Yes, the treatment sounds less than appealing but it is performed under local anaesthetic and as the laser is set on a wavelength that would only affect the vein, the surrounding skin is left unharmed.
- **Sclerotherapy**: This is a simple, anaesthetic-free way to deal with spider veins. A chemical called sclerosant is injected into veins, where it then damages the lining of the vein, causing blood to drain from the vein. After the injection, pressure is applied from the outside to the veins to stop blood from returning. It takes between five to thirty minutes, depending on severity and the number of veins being treated. The cons of sclerotherapy are that you may feel burning or cramping in the affected area and that sclerotherapy may need to be repeated more than once.

Rosacea

Rosacea is an auto-inflammatory skin condition, which means it is caused by a malfunction in the body's defence mechanisms.

You may have rosacea if you have flushing redness on your face that appears to get worse after being in the sun, wind or cold, after drinking alcohol, or after eating spicy food, though not everyone will notice this. If the redness stays the same all the time, it may just be high redness or high colouring which can be genetic – a bit of rosiness in your cheeks that remains all year round and rarely changes.

There are four main types of rosacea:

- **Erythematotelangiectatic rosacea**: This is the type of rosacea I see the most of by far. In appearance, it manifests as flushing and

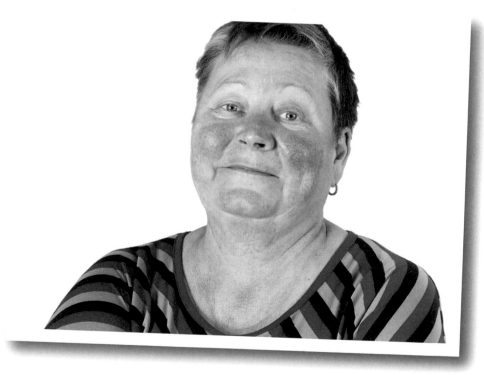

redness as well as small blood vessels becoming visible through the skin. From a symptom perspective, the affected area may sting, burn or become rough.

- **Papulopustular rosacea**: Some refer to this as 'acne rosacea' as it features papules and pustules, just like in acne. In this type of rosacea, there will also be redness, swelling of the skin and plaques (risen, red patches on the skin when the surrounding skin is not affected).
- **Phymatous rosacea**: The skin will become thicker and the texture may be irregular and have nodules or bumps. Phymatous rosacea can often be found on the nose, possibly leading to rhinophyma, which is a bulbousness of the tip of the nose.
- **Ocular rosacea**: This is rosacea of the eyes, where the eyes may become red and irritated and may develop sty-like lumps.

The exact cause of rosacea is still unknown – even when it comes to knowing who is most likely to get rosacea, we have to work on observation. It's been observed that those of Celtic heritage are prone to rosacea (no surprise there, what aren't we prone to?). Interestingly, rosacea is more common in women, but men are more likely to have severe rosacea. Rosacea is also linked to your genes but often doesn't appear fully until middle age. Menopause can trigger rosacea in women too, as if they don't have enough to deal with!

Recent research has discovered a link between rosacea and a little creature called the demodex mite. This may sound like a creepy-crawly but it most certainly is not and is actually a normal and important inhabitant of our skin. The demodex is a type of microbe that gobbles up dead skin cells to reduce waste on the face – the mite is a bit like one of those robot hoovers, except for your face.

How many demodex are found on the skin of those with rosacea? Sometimes up to fifteen to eighteen times as many as on those without rosacea. There is a common agreement is that the excess presence of this mite is to blame for rosacea. Dr Fabienne Forton, a Belgian dermatologist, certainly believes this, as when the amount of mites were normalised during a study in which he was involved, the sufferers no longer complained of skin sensitivity.

Rosacea treatments

- Knowing your triggers is key and they should, obviously, be avoided wherever possible. If drinking is a trigger, cut down or be aware that you're not helping yourself.
- Vitamin C is fabulous as it helps strengthen capillaries and bring down redness, both topically and when ingested.
- Avoid acids and anything that can sensitise your skin – you want to keep your pH where it is.
- Hyaluronic acid, not being like the other acids, is a great hydrator for skin with rosacea.
- The positive effect of omegas on inflammation means that they are key for rosacea as it is simply inflammation.
- Soothers such as green tea extract and liquorice-root extract (like in IMAGE's Iluma serum) should be in your routine too as they will calm and cool where possible.
- If you get heat off your rosacea, pop a hydrating spritz in the fridge and Spritz O'Clock throughout your flare-up. This will keep the skin from become dehydrated and will be more refreshing than an ice-cream cone.
- Probiotics internally can help with inflammation so they are a must-have for those with inflammation-related concerns like rosacea and eczema.
- Vitamin A can attempt to repair the skin at a cellular level which is key in this scenario.

Eczema (Dermatitis)

Eczema (which can also be called dermatitis) usually presents itself as itchy, inflamed, swollen and crusty patches of skin. Like rosacea, the exact cause of eczema is unknown but it is thought to be linked to the body having too severe a response to something that is irritating the immune system.

Eczema is a lifelong skin condition but it may wax and wane. At some point in life, you may not have eczema symptoms for years until a bout of serious stress and then it could disappear just as fast.

It's a wound. It's the cell turnover occurring too quickly in one area which means the skin is more open to the elements. Traditionally, emollient and fat-based ingredients are given to provide temporary relief – they will relieve itching and pain in the area but they don't address the root of the issue.

Eczema treatments

- Omegas, omegas, omegas (which are EFAs, remember). People often look baffled when they report their eczema to me and I ask them 'Do you eat nuts? Do you get EFAs in?' Given that omegas strengthen the barrier, they can greatly help with eczema.
- Probiotic skincare is also amazing for eczema as it balances the skin and colonises the bacteria already on it – many find that this eases their eczema phenomenally.
- Creating long-term skin health with hyaluronic acid, antioxidants, vitamins A, C and E, and SPF is key.

Psoriasis

Psoriasis is a genetic, autoimmune disease that is characterised by flare-ups. Psoriasis presents as patches of scaly skin or plaques that often appear when triggered – you may also feel some heat from the skin with psoriasis. Each person with psoriasis has their own individual triggers, and there are no set rules for what will bring on a flare-up. Many find that drinking alcohol and stress can trigger their psoriasis.

Psoriasis may leave skin dry to the point of cracking and bleeding. In the skin of psoriasis sufferers, inflammation in the body leads to their skin overproducing new skin cells. In the process of keratinisation, the body gets rid of old skin cells to make room for new ones, like stocking shelves in a supermarket. With psoriasis, the overproduction of

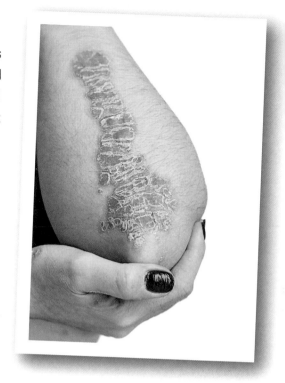

skin cells means that the body has to try to shed off the dead skin cells frantically, but they are just not ready to go. This leaves those skin cells to accumulate on the surface of the skin, forming the plaques of scaly skin.

Psoriasis is typically found on outer parts of the body, such as the elbows.

Psoriasis treatments

- Psoriasis is a medical disorder and for treatment options you should consult your doctor.
- UV therapy has been shown to be effective – seek medical attention to explore this option. (This does not mean sun beds!)
- Omegas, antioxidants, Vitamin A and Vitamin C can help when taken internally too.
- Do not take acids as it could trigger a flare-up (remember, the affected skin is a wound).

- Probiotic skincare can also help. Keeping the skin hydrated, moisturised and protected is so important when it comes to psoriasis. Take internal probiotics for inflammation too.

Eczema versus psoriasis

Because they present in such a similar way, it is really important that you speak to your GP and have a proper diagnosis. They are different in origin. Many believe eczema to be caused by a defective skin barrier but it is often said that it may be related to immune system responses, just like psoriasis.

Accelerated Ageing

Ageing is inevitable but some people look much older than their years – they may only be in their thirties but will look like they're in their forties. Ageing is not a concern but accelerated ageing is.

Compare yourself to your peers – genetics and ethnicity will have a large role – but if your have any of the following, you may be dealing with accelerated ageing:

- Your lines and creases are deeper.
- Your nasolabial (folds to either side of the nose) is deeper.
- Your jawline less defined.
- Your frown lines remain furrowed for longer without animation.
- Your skin appears a little bit rougher, redder and discoloured than that of your peers.

Accelerated ageing occurs because of extrinsic factors, including medication. Prevention is easier than treatment in most things, but this is especially true when it comes to accelerated ageing. Go out in the sun less, don't smoke,

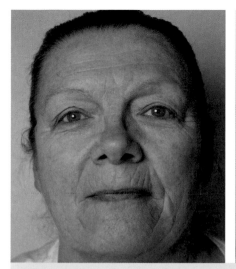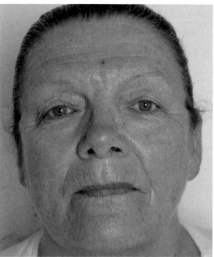

As you can see, the lines around the client's mouth, specifically the nasolabial lines (the ones running between the nose and the mouth) are much less deep than before. The same goes for the lines around her eyes. She is more radiant and her skin looks much healthier.

drink less caffeine, drink alcohol sparingly, bin the wipes and ditch the scrubs. All of these things can be helpful. You should also practise the following:

- Apply topical antioxidants and UV protection daily to stop damage from light and free radicals (which are everywhere).
- Take Vitamin C for internal synthesis of collagen, hyaluronic acid to plump up the skin (more of a temporary solution but hydration is also key) and peptides.
- Use topical Vitamin A, which is just so integral for ageing as it strengthens the skin over time and can heal and prevent pigmentation too, which is associated with ageing skin.

Milia

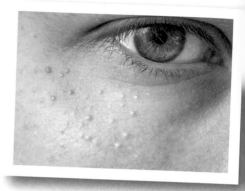

Milia are the small, round, hardened pearly bumps, most often found around the eye area of the face. They look a little bit like a regular whitehead but are visibly deeper in the skin and usually are not accompanied by the ring of redness that a whitehead would have. You are likely to get them in multiples, rather than one milium (yes, that is the word for the singular form). Chances are you've tried to remove them and they wouldn't budge.

Milia are what occurs when sebum and dead skin cells become trapped in the outer layers of the skin. After a while, they keratinise, meaning that they gather keratin (a protein) and then harden. We are not angry at keratin – after all, keratin is an essential structural protein of the skin and looks out for our skin all of the time – it is just that, in this instance, keratin is the culprit of the hardening of these bumps.

There is no 100 per cent foolproof way to prevent milia, but keeping your skin healthy (with EFAs and Vitamin A, in particular) should help as it will prevent the dead skin cells and oil from becoming trapped in the first place. The most effective way to have them removed is the most traditional way – lancing. Go to a salon or clinic and they will pierce the skin with a blade or needle and remove the milium from the skin. Do not try this at home.

Dark Circles

I've spoken to clients who have spent hundreds on lotions and potions (and who have put up with people inferring that they are party animals for years) but who have never been able to kick the circles to the kerb. What many people don't know is that dark circles can be hereditary. They can also appear darker on some people because of the thickness of the skin under the eye. Those with deep-set eyes and thin, periorbital skin (the skin around the orbital bone that surrounds the eye) cannot do a whole lot about the appearance of dark circles.

In the same logic, when you lose the padding around the eye area, the blueness of the veins below shines through and the orbital bone becomes more defined. This creates the hollow of a dark circle. So if you've lost weight, your dark circles will become more pronounced. It's the same if you have mature skin – as your skin becomes thinner with age, your tissue begins to break down.

Your dark circles could also be the result of periorbital hyperpigmentation, which is a darkening of the pigment in the under-eye area and more commonly occurs in those with darker skin tones. It is infamously difficult to treat, usually needing more than one line of attack. It may be genetic, but it can be exacerbated by sun exposure – which is yet *another* reason to apply SPF every bloody day.

Caffeine can boost blood flow underneath the skin to brighten up the area and stop blood from pooling and creating that darkness. Opt for it in a general serum or in a specific eye cream like the SkinCeuticals AOX+ Eye Gel or the Nuxe Crème Prodigieuse Eye Cream.

If your dark circles are pigment-related, the same things apply as they would to any other pigment. Treat them with lighteners and tyrosinase inhibitors, such as Vitamin C and liquorice-root extract like in IMAGE's Iluma Intense Brightening Eye Cream.

In clinics, you can have platelet-rich plasma treatment done (PRP for short), otherwise known as the vampire facial. In PRP, your own blood is taken, the plasma within it separated from the rest in a special machine, and it is then injected back into your skin. This gives the skin growth factors and puts it in 'healing mode' because of the mild trauma of injection, so that fresh skin is created at a rapid pace. This is more suitable for those who have hereditary dark circles like myself. I have received this treatment and rave about it.

With pigment-related dark circles, IPL (intense pulsed light) treatment could be beneficial. The wavelengths target the pigment and bring it to the surface of the skin to flake off.

Blocked Pores

Blocked pores are caused by sebum, which fills the pore and enlarges it. The pore itself has to hold this plug for a while and this will make it less elastic in general, less able to snap back (like a rubber band that has been put around a watermelon repeatedly) and thus an open pore forms.

As we age, our skin becomes less elastic anyway because of degradation and less making of elastin, so this can exacerbate the problem.

Try these treatments for blocked pores:
- Pores must be unclogged of their build up and the elasticity and strength of the pores must be restored and then maintained. You'll need an acid of some sort to do this, dependent on other factors of your skin. If you are spot-prone and quite oily, salicylic acid will do the trick – this should work for most with open pores as they are usually caused by excessive oiliness.
- Glycolic acid suits other skin types and lactic acid is best for a slightly more reactive skin that needs more moisture.
- Poly-hydroxy acid is fabulous for those with a semi-reactive skin.
- If your skin truly can't handle acids (skin is noticeably more tender and touch-sensitive), look into enzymatic exfoliation (good enzymes, not enzymes that can get in and destroy your collagen and elastin, so don't worry).
- The next step is improving the health of each individual pore. Vitamin A is the man for this, specifically Environ's Skin EssentiA AVST step-up programme. It gets to the point that when you're on this fourth step, you have to be careful with waxing, which is how tight your pores get.

- Niacinamide – pop quiz: can you remember which vitamin that is? – is similarly known for improving the appearance of pores when applied topically, so something that includes this could be perfect alongside the others.

Dilated/Open Pores

Normal pores should be no larger than the tip of a safety pin (i.e. visible upon inspection but not something you'll see from arm's-length).

Pore size does vary with ethnicity and heat (which will cause pores to dilate – FYI, they never actually close). Pores are hard to treat if they are bothering you. They can appear bigger as a result of mechanical pulling of the skin (i.e. people poking and prodding and squeezing). Be mindful of this and do your best to stop.

Most often, we struggle with our pores as a result of depleting elasticity levels in the skin. Because of this, the pore has lost its tight disposition – I always imagine it like a new elastic band versus an overused one, one springs back and one, erm, needs a bit of TLC!

For large pores, step away from the blackhead strips and the toners that claim to close them (Lord, give me strength). Instead, keep your pores in check with SPF and Vitamin A. SPF is key as this prevents too much light getting into the dermal layer where the elastin lives – too much sunlight will cause the elasticity to break down and become slackened and so more pores are probable. Vitamin A triggers elasticity within the skin, right at the layer where the elastin is breaking down. Apply this topically and get it through your diet and supplements. Add in clinic microneedling as well as this also triggers elasticity.

Melasma

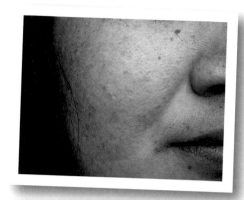

Melasma, which we've already touched upon, is pigmentation triggered by internal hormonal fluctuations, most typically associated with pregnancy. It presents in a 'butterfly' fashion across the forehead, cheek or nose region.

Melasma patches will be one to two shades darker than your natural skin tone and look slightly tea-stained, or like a tan that only hit a certain part of your face.

It is difficult to prevent melasma from worsening as we cannot always nip it in the bud internally. Some women get it during the menopause, which is hardly something we are looking to stop just to prevent melasma. Melasma can be treated in the same way as any other pigmentation, with patience and no promise of curing.

To treat melasma try the following:

- Speak to your GP as it is often related to hormones – it can also be triggered by pregnancy – and some find they get it while on some forms of birth control, such as certain pills, the IUD or the implant bar.
- Wear your SPF. Wear enough of it, wear a high enough factor and top it up. Melasma gets worse with sun exposure – fact. It has to be broad spectrum too, it can't just be UVB protection. Seeing as it is a type of pigmentation, from an aesthetician standpoint, we treat it the same way.
- A lightening serum, such as one that contains Vitamin C or kojic acid, can do wonders and everyday antioxidant protection, which will usually also be provided by a lightening serum, is key.
- Ultimately, as melasma is an internal hormonal inflammation, it needs to be dealt with internally (i.e. if you are on a birth control pill or a specific medication, we cannot 'fix' it topically as the ammunition is being taken

daily on the inside.) This is a conversation to have with your doctor.

- Topical Vitamin A will help to repair the DNA of melanocyte cells and hence will help with any pigment-related condition.
- I don't believe in aciding-off pigmentation as many skincare professionals do. It doesn't actually treat the problem; it just gets that pigment to slough off over time and this can leave you more photosensitive too. It is light that triggers the issue so I often feel it is counter-productive.
- Vitamin A helps with exfoliation as does ascorbic acid, the purest form of Vitamin C.

Hyperpigmentation

We've already discussed both hyperpigmentation and hypopigmentation (see pages 96–98). UV rays are a big reason that many people get hyperpigmentation, as they trigger the creation of melanin. Melanin is our skin's own way of protecting us from UV damage but it can only do so much. Climates have changed and our inherent mode of sun protection can no longer act effectively. UV rays can also damage the melanocyte cell itself, leading to long-term pigmentation problems and, sometimes, skin cancer.

There's also post-inflammatory hyperpigmentation (PIH), which occurs at the site of trauma or injury to the skin – basically, anywhere there has been inflammation. This is why scars and marks can be darker and why people with acne can be left with purple, red or brown patches even after their acne is no longer active. The inflammation can cause damage to the DNA of skin cells, which can bring on the production of melanin.

Wearing perfume directly on your skin can make the skin photosensitive and thus more susceptible to the formation of hyperpigmentation. This is why some people may notice a perfume-drip shaped patch of lighter (hypopigmented) or darker (hyperpigmented) skin behind their ears, on their neck or on their wrists, depending on where they wear it. This doesn't

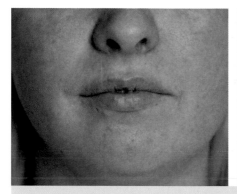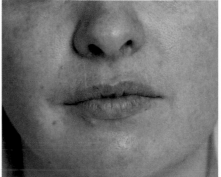

This client is six weeks into her programme for pigmentation. When you first start targeting pigment marks, they may worsen as they move up through the layers of the skin towards the surface and this is what you're seeing in the second image. As you can see, her skin tone is much more even and brighter and the redness around her nose has improved.

mean you have to ditch your fragrance or go around being smelly. Spray your perfume on your clothes instead of on your person – I have it on good authority that it does mean that the perfume doesn't mingle with your skin's natural oils and scents to adapt to you, but it's small price to pay, in my opinion.

Medications can also be the cause of hyperpigmentation. This form is known simply as drug-induced pigmentation, and it's a known side-effect of using certain anti-malaria medication for a longer period of time.

An enzyme called tyrosinase is partially responsible for deciding how much melanin our bodies create so we tackle pigmentation with ingredients known as tyrosinase inhibitors. As you can probably guess from the name, it stops tyrosinase from getting where it needs to go to trigger the production of melanin – et voilà, bye, bye, pigment. This is highly effective as a method of prevention and maintenance of the pigment but we also need to take other steps to prevent and different ones to correct. I am reluctant to say it ever goes permanently.

Vitamin C is particularly beneficial to those with pigmentation as it can lighten it. Some forms are also potent tyrosinase inhibitors.

Vitamin A can help to repair the DNA of skin cells, including melanocyte cells, so getting this on topically is essential when it comes to treating pigment.

Exfoliation will help to bring pigment up through the layers of the skin but you shouldn't skip the other steps and shoot straight to acids. Exfoliation should happen alongside the other treatments that are bringing the cells to health and preventing more pigment from forming, rather than in lieu of it. Glycolic acid is often thought of when it comes to pigmentation but other acids will do the trick too. Be cautious though, as acids make the skin more light-sensitive so you need to be really vigilant when it comes to your sunscreen so that you don't open the skin up to more pigmentation forming.

Like everything, sunscreen is also key, and should always broad spectrum. With pigmentation, use factor 50. Don't risk it for the sake of getting a bit of a colour, as you may get a whole lot of colour you didn't expect, giving you a little pigment moustache.

For intense, widespread light-related hyperpigmentation or acne-related pigmentation, a course of peels designed for pigmentation can be really beneficial for some.

Sun Damage

A lot of people who have pale Celtic skin would love a darker skin tone because we've been conditioned by the media in the Western world to associate a tan with wealth and health. In reality, it's best to stick to the natural colour of your skin, whatever that is. If you're naturally very pale, the only healthy way to get a tan is to fake it.

Sunbeds are *not* the answer. They are a synthetic light at close proximity and are known to be a cause of skin cancer. I have interviewed many people who used them, or who had loved ones who used them and, as a result, had basal cell carcinoma (cancerous growths or lesions that come about in the skin's basal layer) removed, leaving lifelong scars and memories – and, sometimes, led to more serious illness.

Yes, Vitamin D is needed and sunlight is key for many health reasons beyond skincare, however, basting ourselves with oil like a Christmas turkey to bake in the sun is immature and irresponsible, given what we know now about the sun and ageing.

There are three rays that we're exposed to from the sun: UVA, UVB and UVC. C is predominantly protected by the ozone layer; B is only present where the sun shines (think B for burn). A rays are the longest (and we're exposed to them all year round even when it's cold) so penetrate into the living deeper layers of the skin causing accelerated ageing. These are deadly rays.

Shielding the skin is key but it is virtually impossible to cover every single centimetre of your body with sunscreen so that no sun can touch you at all. All you need is for the sun to hit any exposed area of skin for Vitamin D to be synthesised and you get enough in a twenty-minute period. Be safe in the sun and don't lie to yourself – you don't need that much Vitamin D, you just want a tan – and a tan is *always* a sign of sun-related skin damage.

Sun damage (aka photodamage) is seen in age spots, discolouration, redness, freckles, loss of elasticity, lines, white marks (hypopigment) and, yes, a tan. Although we celebrate it, we are not born with the tan and should recognise that it's the body's way of defending itself. It's a sign that your skin has been damaged. If you are born with pigment in your skin, this is not a tan, this is your genetic makeup. The other extreme is having kids so protected that they fear the sun – an educated balance is ideal.

The Most Important Skingredients

In this chapter, we will explore my favourite skingredients, some of which you'll already be familiar with from the Nutrition chapter (see page 49). I've broken these down in terms of acids, antioxidants, hydrators and lightening (which is the term used in skincare for brightening and correcting skin colour) ingredients.

Acids

Glycolic acid

Glycolic acid is probably the most commonly used AHA (alpha-hydroxy acid). It is the smallest AHA molecule, which means it can penetrate deeper into the skin than its cousins, lactic acid, mandelic acid and citric acid. Because of this, it is not as easily controlled and can cause huge change very quickly. This is a double-edged sword as it is also slightly more likely to cause irritation. Glycolic acid, like all AHAs, gets into the skin and prompts the dead skin cells on the upper layers to slough themselves off. This constant cell turnover means that it can dehydrate the skin and is best used alongside hydrating ingredients.

Overuse of glycolic acid can be detrimental to the skin, hence the importance of long-term guidance alongside its usage. Glycolic acid is derived from sugar cane – don't use sugar to exfoliate unless it is chemically with glycolic acid! A word to the spot-prone: some find it brings up an abundance of under-the-surface buggers.

For a good glycolic range, I like the IMAGE Ageless range, particularly the cleanser and serum and overnight mask.

Helps with: Ageing skin, dull skin, those looking to get rid of pigment, sluggish skin, hardier skin.

Be conscious of: If you're dealing with breakouts glycolic acid can bring things to the surface and cause your skin to purge.

Lactic acid

Lactic acid is possibly the reason why Cleopatra bathed in milk! It was first found in sour milk but it can also be synthesised (in this case, made in a lab to mimic the effect of milk-derived formats). It is an AHA like glycolic acid but it is a much larger molecule, which means that it works more slowly and is therefore more gentle, yet effective. Lactic acid is the acid to go for if you have more reactive skin.

In smaller doses, lactic acid can also hydrate the skin by preventing transepidermal water loss. Lactic acid molecules, although larger than glycolic acid ones, still get down deep enough to speed up cell turnover so it will be nearly as effective on hyperpigmentation, dullness and fine lines. Due to the strength and potency of glycolic acid, lactic acid is often considered safer to use during pregnancy.

The best lactic acid I could recommend is Environ derma-lac, for all over the body product and face. It's great for keratosis pilaris which we'll discuss in the Full Body Skin chapter (page 257).

Helps with: Sensitive skin, ageing skin, acne-prone skin, pigment, dull skin, sluggish skin.

Be conscious of: If your skin is particularly sensitive to all acids, or you've had a reaction before to a similar acid, then you should patch test.

Salicylic acid

Salicylic acid is also known as beta-hydroxy acid (BHA) and is derived from willow bark. It is *the* chemical exfoliant for oily and acne-prone skin, as it penetrates into the pore and dissolves the plug of dead skin cells and oils. Salicylic acid also prompts the skin to slough off skin cells from the top, just as AHAs do, but it is gentler as it is anti-inflammatory in nature.

It is thought that salicylic acid works on any lumps and bumps, including keratosis pilaris and ingrown hairs, as these are caused by a fault in the skin's keratinisation process where the skin does not fully shed off dead skin cells and they become stuck in the pore. Note that studies have shown that oral salicylic acid (aspirin) in high doses may not be safe during pregnancy.

My favourite salicylic range is the IMAGE Clear Cell.

Helps with: Oily, spot-prone skin, keratosis pilaris, post-waxing or shaving, bacne, bum spots, those who work out and build up a sweat.

Be conscious of: Don't use during pregnancy. Don't overuse it and if you are allergic to aspirin don't use it as they both derive from the same ingredients (aspirin is properly named as acetylsalicylic acid).

Polyhydroxy acids

Polyhydroxy acids are not a skingredient in themselves, they're more a subcategory of acids. You've got your AHAs, BHA and then you also have PHAs. Polyhydroxy acids are basically just like AHAs except that they are more suitable for reactive skins and those with inflammatory skin conditions.

Two well-known polyhydroxy acids are gluconolactone, a free-radical scavenger, and lactobionic acid, which reduces the appearance of hyperpigmentation and hydrates the skin.

With PHAs, you get all the benefits of AHAs (and BHA), such as increased cell turnover and hydration, but they're more gentle. This is because they can't quite penetrate as deeply into the skin as an AHA.

For PHAs, I recommend the Neostrata Bionic Lotion.

Helps with: Those who are a bit sensitive to acids like glycolic or lactic.

Be conscious of: As with all acids, be careful of using them on broken skin.

Antioxidants

Green-tea extract

Green-tea extract, (EGCG, epigallocatechin gallate or camellia sinensis) is one of the most well-researched antioxidant ingredients and you will find it in the majority of skin-lightening (brightening) products as well as pollution-protective products. Green tea is full of polyphenols, structures that hunt down free radicals. Free-radical damage leads to premature ageing so this is a good type of hunt!

Green-tea extract is also soothing, because of the anti-inflammatory nature of polyphenols, which means it can be helpful with inflammatory skin conditions and helps to bring down redness and irritation. Green tea itself is also beneficial as a beverage as it has very similar effects from the inside out – the perfect alternative to tea and coffee as the polyphenols make up for the high caffeine content. Just a note: rubbing your face with a wet green tea bag will not work! If you're looking for green-tea extract to apply topically, go for IMAGE Ormedic Bio Peptide Serum.

Helps with: those looking for antioxidant protection as well as soothing of redness.

Be conscious of: Make sure you don't have an allergy to green tea!

Coenzyme Q10

Coenzyme Q10 (ubiquinol, Co-Q10 or ubiquinol) is a chemical compound. It is used in skincare primarily for its antioxidant properties as it is another free-radical scavenger. This coenzyme is a game-changer. It's the final element in the energy chain, and is a youth booster to both bodies and skin, heading straight into the cell's mitochondria ('engine room') to generate cellular energy. Additionally, it aids in the growth of cells to minimise the appearance of fine lines.

Coenzyme Q10 is something your body knows very well because it exists within your cells but as we age, our natural production of Co-Q10 slows down dramatically. You can find Co-Q10 in both topical and ingestible formulations and it is shown to reduce the signs of ageing when taken in a supplement. It is a fab skingredient to add to your routine to defend from pollution-related damage.

For Coenzyme Q10, I would recommend Dermastir Coenzyme Q10 Twisters and Trilogy CoQ10 Booster Oil.

Helps with: Someone looking to tackle the signs of ageing hard whilst getting antioxidant protection.

Be conscious of: There's little to be conscious of here unless you have a known allergy to this ingredient, which is rare.

Resveratrol

Resveratrol is something we covered in the Nutrition chapter (see page 49), but it's also something you'll find in products.

It's a phytonutrient, specifically a polyphenol, that acts as an antioxidant itself and also boosts the body's own supply of enzymes that battle free-radical damage. Resveratrol, like all antioxidants, battles the free

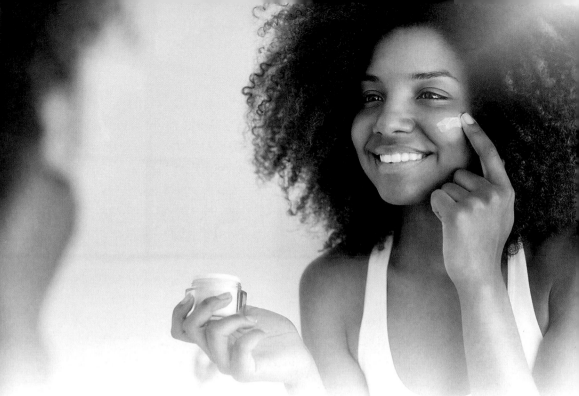

radicals that cause premature ageing but it is also possible that it inhibits tyrosinase, the enzyme that causes the formation of pigmentation in the skin. Taking this on the inside wins out but for a good topical option, try SkinCeuticals Resveratrol CE.

Helps with: Protecting from pollution-related ageing when used topically because of its free-radical scavenging nature.

Be conscious of: As this is a plant derived antioxidant there should be no issues.

Hydrators

Hyaluronic acid

This acid is not like the others, hence why it is here in hydrators!

When people see acid, they presume exfoliation of some form but hyaluronic acid is not an exfoliant, it is a hydrator extraordinaire. Our body makes hyaluronic acid itself but, as we get older, this production slows down, which is one of the reasons why skin becomes less hydrated and more crêpe-like as the years go by.

Hyaluronic acid can hold up to a thousand times its weight in water and it is a humectant (it draws water towards it). When applied topically, it pulls water upwards from the lower layers of the skin, instantly plumping out and hydrating the uppermost layers. This makes it not so ideal for times when your skin is already dehydrated or your skin's barrier function is impaired, as it can just dehydrate the skin further by bringing the moisture right out of the skin.

Different forms of hyaluronic acids have different molecular sizes, which means they can get into different depths within the skin depending on what you're looking for. Sodium hyaluronate, the salt of hyaluronic acid, can come in smaller molecular size to pure hyaluronic acid and therefore can get further down into the layers of the skin.

For this I turn to Pestle + Mortar Hyaluronic Serum. It is a hydration boost – a slick of moisture.

Helps with: The summer months when there is high humidity. Those with dehydrated skin, dry skin, acne-prone skin (hydrates without oiliness or heaviness) – everyone really.

Be conscious of: As it's a humectant, it can draw a lack of hydration into the skin, so if you find yourself in very dry conditions (e.g. winter, aeroplanes, hot desert), avoid use for a while.

Squalane

Squalane, with an *a*, is saturated form of squalene, with an e. This means that it is squalene that has been hydrogenated. The hydrogenation process stabilises the squalene and makes it last longer, as squalene 'goes off' very quickly. Squalene is a compound found in the skin's sebum. It is one of the most natural skingredients you'll find as it is actually native to the skin. As an oil, it is fabulous for those with dry, dehydrated or mature skin as these are the type of skins that aren't producing a lot of squalene themselves.

It is non-comedogenic, meaning it doesn't clog pores, and has antibacterial qualities. One noteworthy thing about squalane is that it takes a while to absorb into the skin. When it is a secondary ingredient in skincare, this slow absorption is negated by the penetrant enhancing ingredients.

My favourite squalane product range is Doctor Jart Ceramidin.

Helps with: Dry skin, dehydrated skin and mature skin.

Be conscious of: If you're a vegetarian or vegan make sure the squalane product is plant derived as opposed to animal derived.

Vitamins

Vitamin A

Vitamin A is the only vitamin that can cause a physical change within the skin and repair DNA damage – can I get an A-men? We believe that Vitamin A is the first building block to skin health and that everyone should be getting it both topically through a serum and internally through supplements – unless you are pregnant or breastfeeding, when it comes to ingestion!

I have lectured alongside doctors and nurses who will argue black is white and white is black *but* they all agree this ingredient is key.

There are many forms of Vitamin A in topical skincare: retinoic acid (aka prescription Vitamin A), retinol (which transforms into retinoic acid within the skin) and retinyl palmitate (which is slightly less irritating to the skin and more stable than retinol). There is also beta-carotene, the form of Vitamin A that gives plants and vegetables such as carrots an orange colour and what your parents told you gave you night vision.

Our Nerdie choice is usually retinyl palmitate in a progressive product, which means it is introduced slowly and surely, rather than firing a more active form on the skin that can only be used intermittently – it's a lot like starting with small weights at the gym before adding more as you go, rather than going in on day one expecting yourself to lift 20kg without doing yourself harm. This is because its stability and bioavailability means that it is less likely to cause a retinoid response (i.e. Vitamin A-related skin irritation). Interestingly, if you apply retinol, it converts back into retinyl palmitate first to be absorbed.

My favourite progressive Vitamin A product is Environ AVST. You start with AVST 1 and when your skin is used to that, you go up to AVST 2, etc.

Helps with: It's a general building block of skin health that everyone needs.

Be conscious of: Don't use if you are pregnant (unless you specifically use Environ AVST 1 or 2 which they advise is safe during pregnancy). If you are breastfeeding, only use a topical version but do check before using as only certain doses are allowed.

Vitamin C

Vitamin C is key, as it's not something we make naturally. Vitamin C has so many fabulous benefits: it can strengthen capillary walls (preventing broken capillaries and diffused redness), it is integral to the skin's synthesis of collagen and it is an antioxidant and so can battle pollution-related damage. It

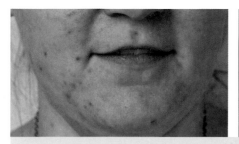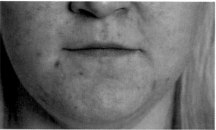

This client was concerned with her post-spot redness (aka post-inflammatory hyperpigmentation) and the clarity, radiance and immunity of her skin is now apparent. Her spots are still occurring, although less often and smaller, and she isn't left with as much PIH as a reminder of them. We advised her to introduce Vitamin C to her routine – by taking supplements and applying the Neostrata Enlighten Illuminating Serum (which contains some Vitamin C).

is also a tyrosinase inhibitor, meaning that it stops the enzyme that produces melanin from overproducing it and causing pigmentation problems.

The purest form of Vitamin C is l-ascorbic acid which, unfortunately, is only at its most effective within ten days of exposing it to any air at all but it is highly potent: even with this drop in efficacy, it will still contain higher levels of Vitamin C than many other products!

Other forms of Vitamin C in topical products include ascorbyl tetraisopalmitate (oil-soluble so fab at penetrating), magnesium ascorbyl phosphate (water-soluble and highly stable), retinyl ascorbate (a mix of retinoic acid, aka Vitamin A, and ascorbic acid) and tetrahexyldecyl ascorbate (a highly stable form that works well with other forms of Vitamin C).

Each form of Vitamin C works best in different formulations, dependent on the other ingredients and what type of product it is.

Helps with: Those looking to tackle pigmentation, synthesise more collagen and antioxidise. Particularly good for its anti-ageing qualities.

Be conscious of: *If you are very congested avoid Vitamin C in its purest form (L-ascorbic acid) as it can irritate congestion-prone skin.*

Vitamin E

Vitamin E is best known as a highly potent antioxidant that can protect the skin from UVA damage. It is lipophilic, meaning it is oil-soluble, and thus can boost the skin's hydration. There are many forms of Vitamin E in skincare but alpha-tocopherol is thought to be the most useful to human skin as it is highly biologically active. Alpha-tocopherol can come in both synthetic and natural form, but the natural form has been proven to be more effective.

Vitamin E has been put to use for its moisturising properties for decades, so it is also ideal as an additional source of skin hydration. Be wary, though, Vitamin E can be slightly comedogenic and so can bring on congestion in those with naturally oilier skin. Vitamin E is perfect for those with dehydrated, dry or mature skin because of its softening and moisturising effects. For a good Vitamin E product, I would recommend Skinceuticals CE Ferulic, IMAGE Vital C Hydrating Antioxidant A C E Serum, Yon-Ka Vital Defense, Académie Sun Stick Sensitive Areas SPF 50+ and Environ AVST 1-5.

Helps with: Most skin types, dehydrated skin, dry, skin and mature skin.

Be conscious of: Those with very oily or congestion-prone skin should only use it in small doses.

Peptides

Peptides are two or more amino acids holding hands! They are like protein jigsaw pieces bcause, when some of them link up, they form different types of proteins. Peptides occur naturally in the skin but there are benefits to introducing some more. In skincare products, peptides are used as a backup dancer for your skin's protein, making the whole show a lot stronger.

Peptides can send signals to the dermis to do a number of different things, including upping collagen production, making them a key anti-ageing ingredient. There are more peptides out there in the world than you could imagine, and we still don't know all we can know about them! You will most commonly see peptides in a blend or in the form of copper peptides. No peptide is 'better' than another, they just have different talents.

Peptide products I like include Neostrata Skin Active Firming Collagen Booster, Environ Youth EssentiA Vita Peptide Eye Gel, IMAGE Ormedic Balancing Bio-Peptide Creme, (for men) Académie Scientifique De Beauté Men Active Stimulating Balm for Deep Lines and No7 Lift & Luminate Triple Action Serum.

Helps with: Ageing skin.

Be conscious of: Some (not all) peptides come from soy or rice so if you are allergic to these foods, you're best to avoid these ones. If you are allergic to amino acids, skip peptides.

Lightening Ingredients

By 'lightening' ingredients and products, I don't mean ingredients that will make dark skin appear more white or white skin appear more pale – it's all about brightening the skin, addressing discolouration and giving you an even skin tone.

Kojic acid

Kojic acid is fungus for your face, as it is a natural product of fungi. Kojic acid is a tyrosinase inhibitor, meaning that it stops tyrosinase (an enzyme that tells the skin to create melanin) in its tracks. You'll find kojic acid in products that target pigmentation, whether it be post-inflammatory hyperpigmentation (aka acne marks or age spots).

Kojic acid is possibly the ingredient closest to hydroquinone (a highly potent lightening agent that is often banned) but a much safer option, available in Europe and less likely to cause irritation. Hydroquinone can be obtained on prescription and is more readily available in America, it should be used with caution and care.

Product wise, for Kojic acid I recommend Neostrata Enlighten Pigment Lightening Gel.

Helps with: Lightening, pigmentation

Be conscious of: Sometimes, it's derived trom mushrooms (where it was originally found), so if you have a mushroom allergy, be mindful.

Liquorice root extract

Liquorice-root extract is a skin lightener. It's also known as *glycyrrhiza uralensis*, *glycyrrhiza inflate* or *glycyrrhiza glabra* – but 'liquorice root' extract is much easier to say and spell.

Liquorice-root extract is both a tyrosinase inhibitor and a pigment synthesis inhibitor, which means it stops the creation of pigmentation by putting a halt to the pigment-creating enzyme (tyrosinase).

We probably don't need to mention where it comes from but in case you didn't realise, it is extracted from liquorice. Not only does it help to lighten pigmentation and prevent pigmentation problems, such as hyperpigmentation; it is also antioxidant in nature. Antioxidants are what protect your skin from free-radical damage and the related accelerated ageing so it's a fabulous added benefit for liquorice root extract to have. Great products with this skingredient include IMAGE Iluma Intense Lightening Serum and Académie Aromatherapy Treatment Oil For Redness.

Helps with: Soothing, skin brightening, lightening, radiance boosting.

Be conscious of: Allergies to liquorice.

Niacinamide

Niacinamide (Vitamin B3) is a water-soluble vitamin that is proven to help inhibit the transfer of melanosomes (melanin granules that protect the 'mother cell') within the skin. In English, it stops one of the processes that enables hyperpigmentation to form, meaning age spots and acne marks. As well as this, it was shown in studies to increase the brightness of the skin.

It is also shown to help with congestion and the structure of the skin, so can prevent the formation and help the appearance of fine lines and wrinkles. It really is a busy B of a vitamin! For a good Niacinamide product, go for Murad Rapid Age Spot Correcting Serum.

Best for: Skin lightening, pigmentation, skin smoothing, uneven skin tone, has a temporary positive effect on large pores.

The best of the natural skingredients:

Coconut oil
Used as a pre-cleanse, moisturising, it contains vitamins, natural humectant

Jojoba oil
Natural moisturising ingredient from the jojoba plant, hydrating, packed with vitamins and minerals, perfect for really, really sensitive skins

Evening primrose oil
Fabulous for inflammation and acts as an emollient to trap moisture into the skin so it is beneficial to those with drier skin, eczema and psoriasis. It also contains essential fatty acids (EFAs)!

Aloe vera

Great hydrator and highly soothing

Lavender

Healing and energising but can be sensitising

An overview of skincare products to avoid:

- Gritty scrubs – they are too harsh on the skin and may increase sensitivity.
- Eye creams that are indeed cheek creams (i.e. not suitable for use in direct, under-eye area) because they don't serve any purpose for the eye area and you're wasting your money.
- Fad-based masks: Peel-off masks that practically peel your face off and give you a face wax in the process. The black charcoal masks are a no-no.
- Pore strips: These are not stripping your pores, they are cleaning sebaceous filaments. They don't resolve the skin problems, so your blackheads will be back sooner than you can spell 'blackhead'. The best way to avoid blackheads is through exfoliation and consistency in your routine.
- Face wipes: You know why I think these are the devil's make-up remover at this stage!
- Moisturisers that are heavy and cannot penetrate your skin. If a moisturiser feels really thick and heavy on your fingers and on your face, it can't properly penetrate your skin. If it stays on your skin after a few minutes and you're left with a sheen of oil or grease, it's too heavy of a moisturiser. Opt for serums that can actually get into your skin due to their smaller molecular size.

- Brands that encourage people to use products from the same line yet have a duplication of the same ingredients. If a brand has an acne range, often it means that every single product contains salicylic acid or tea tree oil. This is no good because as you probably know by now, your skin benefits much more from multiple ingredients to do multiple jobs! This is why I'm fond of the mix and match approach – it means that your skin gets something to treat spots, something to hydrate it, something to protect it from free radical damage and more … not just lots of one or two ingredients.

Skin Diary Check-in:

Take a look at the above list of ingredients and make note of the ones you think will address your current concerns.

Check the ingredients lists on the products you currently use – the one on the back, not the front. Ingredient potency is listed from the top, left to right. Are your products truly doing what you need them to do?

Cosmeceutical Versus Over-the-counter Products

Understanding the difference between cosmeceutical products and over-the-counter products (OTC) is key when it comes to choosing the right goodies for you and your skin.

Cosmeceutical is a combination of the words 'cosmetic' and 'pharmaceutical'. It's kind of a marketing buzzword more than anything, but a great descriptor nonetheless. If a product is cosmeceutical, it contains enough active ingredients that penetrate into the lower layers of the skin to create changes, for example, tackling bacteria or stimulate collagen. A true cosmeceutical should only be retailed along with the right education and information so that you are aware of how to use it. This is why I am such an advocate of consultations. In a consultation, an expert can impart this knowledge to the client and offer follow-up support. An example of a cosmeceutical product would be one high in glycolic acid, such as IMAGE Skincare's Ageless Total Facial Cleanser.

Over-the-counter products do not contain the amounts of active ingredients that can cause change in the skin. They can be obtained sans consult and without advice. They soothe, pacify and calm the skin and can help boost the skin's barrier function, but it is important to note that not all OTC products are created equal and some can contain harsh and drying fragrances and preservatives.

When buying OTC products, avoid: Large amounts of drying alcohols (listed as denatured alcohol, alcohol denat., SD alcohol), synthetic fragrances listed often as parfum or perfume and large amounts of natural fragrances. It's not so much about individual ingredients - it's about the concentration of them, why they're being used and if the product as a whole is beneficial to the skin.

My experience lies predominantly in the world of the cosmeceutical. I have trained and lectured with brands that began with a plastic surgeon or dermatologist with a dream to spread skin health, such as IMAGE Skincare and Murad. These brands blind test their products and have them tested independently to ensure that the results they are getting are real. For me, the cosmeceutical triumphs over the OTC. They result in long-term measurable changes to the skin.

That said, cosmeceuticals can cause initial irritation, which is why you will always be advised to start small and build up, and they will be more expensive. On top of that, because they are not owned by global beauty brands, they are less accessible (you won't find them in the local supermarket) and you should follow the advice of a consultation to obtain them.

Similarly, there are pros and cons to OTCs. They are affordable, accessible and ideal for immediate effects, such as hydration. I see cosmeceutical skincare as the route for people looking to bring about change in their skin but OTC skincare is ideal for someone maintaining their skin, who wants it to be clean, moist and balanced, but who is not focused on correcting skin concerns.

OTC products I recommend

I like Avène's sunscreens and a bunch of their other products, Gallinée is probiotic skincare that I really like. Neostrata have loads of highly active products all over the counter too – it's a great brand. It is actually a cosmeceutical sold in an OTC manner – I believe this is the future for active skincare. Once education features, I feel it is ethical. No7 is another over the counter brand I like as they use some more cosmeceutically-geared ingredients and make them more accessible for all. For example, many of their newer products contain Matrixyl 3000+, a powerful peptide.

MooGoo is another more pacifying brand that will hydrate, heal and protect the skin and is geared towards people who prefer natural ingredients as it is literally edible. It's fabulous at calming reactive skin and they even have quite a potent Vitamin C serum, so they do dabble in the more active of cosmetic skincare ingredients too.

'Angel Dusting'

It is important to note that many cosmetic skincare brands will do something known as 'angel dusting' so that their ingredients align with massive industry trends.

'Angel dusting' is the term for adding a negligible amount of an active ingredient to a product so that the manufacturer can say the product contains that ingredient. This is a waste of your money as it won't give you the results you need. It is frustrating for therapists like myself and my team because we hear so many clients report they have tried everything – and they believe they have – when actually this isn't the case.

Some more affordable cosmetic products do contain traditionally cosmeceutical-style ingredients and in relatively high levels, but you have to be careful.

I have heard of and seen horror cases where people have overdone it on readily available acids and caused their skin long-term damage. Vitamin C is the type of ingredient that can transition from the cosmeceutical world to the cosmetic world easily. What happens when we have high levels of acids available without a consultation or education? Acids are misused and overused.

Vitamin C in its purest form is ascorbic acid, which will over-exfoliate when it's overused. The fear is that a client will fall in love with a product and overuse it, particularly if they are on a mission or a countdown to an event like a wedding.

This is also seen with acids, such as glycolic acid. In scenarios that are not worst case, I've heard of people breaking out persistently, having flare-ups of lifelong skin conditions and having chronic dry patches because of the unmonitored use of some of products. To avoid irritation or any adverse effects, remember that when it comes to cosmeceuticals, go for a consultation.

In the end, the choice of whether you're using OTC or cosmeceutical skincare is up to you but be cautious when it comes to products offering huge promises without having the research or trials to back it up – you know what they say, if it sounds too good to be true, it probably is!

If you're going for an expensive over-the-counter product that claims to contain an ingredient that will do something really specific for your skin, such as Vitamin C, read the back of the bottle and research the type of

Vitamin C it is, for example. This way, you can tell if it is actually effective and in which amounts.

The only sure way to know you're getting good-quality products and ingredients that will work for your concerns is to have a consultation with a salon, clinic or service that offers many cosmeceutical and cosmetic skincare brands and regularly train with the brands. The training part is essential, as that is where questions like 'What's the percentage of this ingredient?' and 'What does it ACTUALLY do?' get asked.

Natural Versus Chemical Products

When people talk about natural products, they mean products that don't contain chemicals, parabens, alcohol or synthetic fragrances. Natural products will contain botanical and fruit extracts, and, usually, essential oils.

A chemical product is essentially everything else. It's a wobbly line in the sand and nobody has to prove that their product is natural to market it as such – therein lies the problem. You'll often find a product described as natural when it includes some ingredients from natural sources within the product listing.

In my opinion, natural is a term that is overused and perhaps conjures a false image of being 'better than', or 'better for'. Natural ingredients, such as lavender, tea tree and ylang-ylang, have undeniable benefits, and I rate

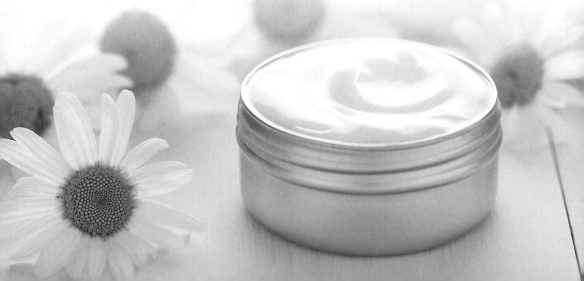

them highly, but are they natural to your skin? Just because something is labelled 'natural' doesn't automatically mean it's the best option.

In my experience, many natural products can also irritate the skin, so it's not only synthetic ingredients that can cause reactions.

Ingredients like witch hazel and tea tree oil have proven skin benefits, but they are very astringent and so can be drying in a high dosage. They also, notably, don't exist in the skin or the body. However, ceramides, squalane, hyaluronic acid, Vitamin A, collagen, amino acid and peptides are naturally found in the skin or the body. So which is truly more natural? In short, don't be put off by chemical-sounding words, and don't be lulled into a false sense of security by things that sound natural.

Something that truly gets my goat is DIY skincare. Many people opt to save money by making skincare at home, such as lemon juice as a pigmentation lightener. The vast majority of homemade skincare hacks do not work. Lemon juice is far too acidic to apply directly to your skin. It is not formulated to ensure that it won't irritate you, and it doesn't have added hydrating ingredients. Popping any old Vitamin C capsule on to your face topically is not the same as using a Vitamin C serum because the molecules will not be small enough to actually penetrate into the epidermis and it is – for the people in the back – not formulated for use on the skin. Yes, pineapple contains enzymes that can exfoliate the skin but, no, this does not mean that you should be rubbing your afternoon snack on your face.

I can't speak for every natural brand out there. There are hundreds of phenomenal natural brands that believe in keeping chemicals to a minimum – MooGoo is one – and that come up with formulas that can soothe the skin. There are also natural brands selling smoothies as serums or claiming their products won't irritate you, when in fact there is always a chance that something could irritate you.

Word to the wise: essential oils irritate many a person's skin worldwide, as do natural ingredients like limonene (a component of citric fruit peels – as in orange peel, not skincare peel).

Also, FYI: Salicylic acid is a derivative of witch hazel, which means it's natural. I am a fan of becoming a skin witch and playing with ingredients, layering masks, doing DIY facials and sprinkling new ingredients into a regime, but I educate myself on the best method.

How long will it be before I see results?

Seeing results depends on the product specifically. For example, pigment spot treatments take longer to work than others (for some brands it could be six months before you see the full results, and this varies from person to person). Usually, it will take twenty-eight days to see measurable changes, two months to see noticeable changes – but this is dependent on the skingredients in the regime, the advice given and whether you're actually doing/using it consistently or not.

How long before I know if something is helping or not?

It actually depends on the type of product. You usually see results from using acids in about one to two weeks, Vitamin C is usually about eight weeks, Vitamin A is between four to eight weeks. You won't see an immediate result from antioxidants but they're protecting you in the future. If you're using a routine for eight weeks and seeing ABSOLUTELY NO result, take a look into what you're using. Patience is important too. This is where your skin diary comes in – take a picture on day one, file it away and assess the difference after a month.

What if things go wrong?

Some products cause something that many call a 'purge'. I don't necessarily believe in purging, but I do believe in the skin reacting to ingredients it hasn't be introduced to yet. Vitamin A is known to cause a 'retinoid reaction'. This may be a bit of redness, dryness and irritation for the initial few weeks of usage as your skin becomes accustomed to it. For some, this manifests as particularly nasty spots. However, time and time again, after two to four weeks of use, this goes away entirely to make way for beautiful, healthy skin. It is similar to a sore muscle after a new workout – your body needs time to adjust.

After using particularly acidic products, such as high-percentage cleansers or at-home peel kits, you may feel a tingle and a teeny tiny bit of a sting. This is relatively normal. If it is anything that you would consider to be even a 0.5 on the pain scale, don't use the product again and speak to whoever sold it to you.

Top tip: other salons or professionals cannot discuss reactions from products that you purchased from a different stockist for insurance reasons, so remember to call your salon or pharmacy first and foremost.

If spots, redness or mild irritation related to a new product doesn't go away in two weeks, speak to your consultant/aesthetician.

When using acids, avoid any broken skin (spots you've picked, cuts, grazes, etc). Also keep them away from your lips because the acids will irritate them.

Product Trends

We will now explore some of the skincare and beauty trends you've no doubt come across, teasing apart the trends worth following and those which you can skip right past.

K-Beauty

Three years ago, K-Beauty was splashed all over *Vogue* and the like but it has now made it into mainstream skincare. Korean skincare enthusiasts are all about essence, double cleansing, sheet masks, snail serums (yes, snails!), spritzing, magnetic masks, quirky brands and novelty skincare.

They are known for their ten to seventeen skincare steps per night and while that might be a lot for you or me, there is a lot we can glean from the K-Beauty regime. I took it upon myself to fly there last year and see for myself. They indeed had more skincare options in the skin capital of Seoul than I could wrap my head around. There were sheet masks to beat the band and I was dizzy from the different options available. I found their love for natural skincare admirable.

Concepts/Steps in Korean Skincare

1. Pre-cleanse
Koreans love an oil cleanse as their pre-cleanse or will use an oil-based balm or fluid for this purpose (as do the Japanese). They oil up the face with their hands in gentle, circular motions and remove it delicately with a warm face cloth.

2. Cleanse
Korean skincare enthusiasts feel strongly that an oil cleanse should be followed with a foaming cleanser. This works because the use of oil in the first steps will stop a potentially drying foam from sapping too much hydration from the skin. A wash or foam will also help to get rid of any makeup or oil traces and treat the skin with whichever actives it contains.

3. Exfoliate
This step is not a daily step for many. Korean people, like myself, understand that daily acid is too much for most people's skin. They exfoliate with a lotion or pre-soaked pad that contains a blend of acids or enzymes between once and three times a week, to keep their cell turnover ticking on and inhibit spots from forming. They, once again like myself, do not like facial scrubs for the most part and they treat their skin with a soft touch.

4. Toners

The Korean concept of a toner is not like the Western one. Our toners can be astringent, acid-packed and drying. Theirs are soothing and hydrating, packed with botanical essences and things like rose water. They also use their toner as a penetrant enhancer to ensure the skin will take in all the lovely skingredients that are yet to come from their serums – now *that* I can get behind.

5. Essences

Essences are a product found in Korean skincare that I believe the rest of the world never really took to. An essence is essentially a more liquid serum or ampoule, or a more concentrated toner. Essences usually contain an ingredient that aids in the skin's cell renewal rate to leave the user with a more even skin tone. You'll often find your typical spot treatment in the form of an essence in a Korean skincare regime which makes more sense – on this side of the planet, many put their spot treatment on either too early or too late in their routine but post-toner and pre-serum is usually where it should be.

6. Serums and boosters

Your serum or booster in a Korean regime is to tackle specific concerns, such as acne, pigmentation, redness or dehydration. They would use it more like a 'treatment' than a hydrator in many circumstances.

7. Masks

We can't talk about K-beauty without mentioning sheet masks. Sheet masks are the preferred mode of masking in a Korean regime and would be used two or three times a week.

Sheet masks, for the uninitiated, are usually a material mask soaked in an intensive serum. The benefit of the sheet is that it works as an

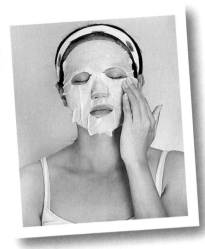

occlusive to lock the product onto the face for the period in which you have the mask on.

Once again, sheet masks are geared towards specific concerns but maybe more for short-term results. For example, in winter, you're more likely to find hydration masques in the cupboards of Korean people, whereas, in summer, you may be more likely to find a clarifying one to tackle any sweat-related congestion.

They also like the 'in a tube' or 'in a tub' mask varieties – it really depends on the individual's skin.

8. Eye creams

Eye creams are, like in Western beauty, for the purpose of tackling dark circles, fine lines and ageing around the eyes. The only difference between Korea and us when it comes to eye cream is that they will use it from a younger age and they won't tug their under eyes when applying it. They believe in tapping it on gently with their ring fingers, which is something we skin therapists also do.

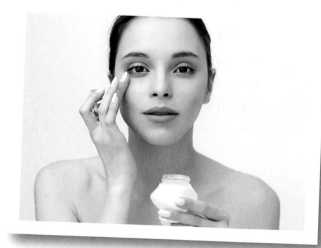

Pulling at the skin can cause mechanical ageing, which is best to avoid.

9. Moisturisers/creams/gels

The purpose of a moisturiser or cream in Korean skincare is for surface-level hydration and to lock in the preceding products like a shield. Personally, I don't believe in a true need for a moisturiser or cream as most serums will contain ingredients that act in the same way.

Oilier-skinned people may opt for a more lightweight consistency for this step, such as a water gel or a cream-gel hybrid.

10. Sunscreen

This is where Korean people have my heart – their undying commitment to protecting their skin from both UVA and UVB rays. Many Korean facial sunscreens are formulated to be easy to wear. They have a pleasant consistency that sinks into the skin well and are perfect for use when occupying a desk job. Most will contain both pollution protection and UV protection.

They're also fans of a tinted SPF as with a skincare regime like this, who needs makeup?

This step is for the morning only, naturally.

Korean application methods

Korean people love a good tap – into their skin that is. They do not rub, pull or tear at their skin. They gently tap their product onto their skin for increased absorption. It's also beneficial for increasing circulation, giving you a nice glow right before you head about your day.

I personally believe in tapping, kneading and knuckling – the muscles in our face are manipulated daily and need relaxing – this is what I do nightly to remove lactic acid from my muscles. It aids relaxation and also helps with 'resting bitch face', if, like me, you are a sufferer.

How to Give Yourself a Facial Massage

Giving yourself a facial massage sounds more difficult than it is. Start by tying back your hair, washing your hands with a cleanser thoroughly (I am not crazy on soaps due to their drying qualities, but I do believe in anti-bacterialising – I'm not a monster) and double-cleansing. You need something to give you a bit of slip to work with – facial oils are the best for this, in my opinion. You can use a natural carrier oil like coconut oil or jojoba oil or a specifically designed facial oil – whatever you like! I adore Urban Veda's facial oils as they smell like a spa and contain amazing botanical ingredients. Alternatively, use a moisturiser – a serum will dry in so you won't get the same slip.

I start from my neck upwards.

Step 1 is to warm your face by gently gliding your palms across it.

Step 2 is to knead your face with the flat part of your finger that you'd wear a ring on. I roll my hand while I do this so that each finger hits the face just a millisecond before the next one.

Step 3 is tapotement, a technique from Swedish massage where you lightly flick the pads of your middle and ring finger in a rolling-upwards motion across the skin. This part shouldn't be with a lot of pressure – it should feel and sound like a flick, as if a butterfly has flown past your ear. It's about rolling your wrists and it should be done quickly.

Step 4 is to warm your face again. You should feel some warmth and see some redness after these steps.

Step 5 We get much more gentle as we're moving on to the eye area. We use our ring fingers here, draining outwards towards the temple with gentle, light, superficial strokes and there should be no tissue movement.

Step 6 I do pressure points. Using the flat of your thumb or your forefinger, NOT the tip, try to find the flat part of the bone about two fingertips away from each nostril. Press in to release facial tension and bring down puffiness – keep doing this all the way along the cheekbone.

Step 7 is to apply your skincare products and go to sleeeeep!

In the morning, I do just the eye bit prior to makeup and when I'm lying in bed, I flick the skin outwards with the pad of my middle finger, as if I'm moving a small wheel or roller ball (like on the bottom of an old school mouse) quickly. This is to get your circulation going and reduce puffiness.

Jade rolling

I use jade stones all the time. Jade stones are a jade-green stone (surprise, surprise) with a smooth surface. All we do with a jade stone is run it over the skin in the direction of lymphatic drainage, towards the heart. Sometimes the stone comes in the form of a roller – the stone will be in the shape of a cylinder on top of a handle and will roll across the skin when you move it.

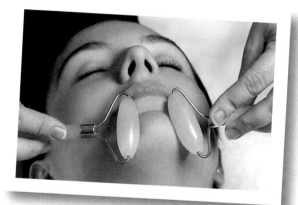

We also jade-stoned the models at London Fashion Week. I personally prefer a full jade stone that fits the facial contour rather than a roller but that's just my preference as it covers more space in one go.

Jade stone works the skin out by promoting lymphatic drainage, which will bring down puffiness across the face and improve blood circulation, which will get you glowing. It is smooth enough not to damage the skin – just make sure to oil (or serum) your face well first and go gently. Work it outwards from the centre of the face to the jawline and do it every day if you can. I can stand behind this one as I see an immediate difference myself. This is a trend that's here to stay.

Charcoal masks

You'll see these all over social media – pictures of influencers, celebrities and your favourite bloggers coated in a sticky gothic black substance – these are charcoal masks. Charcoal, when activated, becomes more porous and gets a larger surface area like an absorbent mini-sponge. It works like a very gentle magnet to 'suck' dirt and debris from the pore. This makes charcoal a worthy skingredient if your masque or product is high in activated charcoal. If it is at the bottom of the ingredient list, give it a miss. And if it's one that you peel off along with the top layer of your skin, AVOID!

I like Seoulista Charcoal Detox Instant Facial. A good charcoal mask will contain lots of activated charcoal (if it's not activated, it doesn't work the same way).

Bubble masks

Bubble masks look and are applied like your traditional clay face mask but within five minutes of wearing them, they become puffy and bubbly, like a fluffy grey cloud across your visage. The way they get them to bubble has to do with a type of ingredient known as perfluorocarbons that can dissolve oxygen gas. In the packaging process, they blast oxygen gas into the mask and lock it into the pressurised packaging. When you apply the mask to your face, the oxygen that was introduced into the mask returns to its gaseous state and causes the bubbles.

Basically, bubble masks introduce some oxygen to the surface of the skin and this improves circulation, bringing nutrients and oxygen to the skin's cells. I said 'some' for a reason – salon or clinic oxygen facials are proven to do this, but bubble masks aren't necessarily.

Like any mask, how beneficial it is depends on the ingredients but it may provide a little extra oomph than a regular mask. It's kind of more of a fun gimmick but skincare is self-care so if you like that gimmick, why not go for it?

There is the issue of oxidation but the low amount of extra oxygen that would be added to the skin maximum once a week (and probably less) probably wouldn't make a huge impact.

At-home LED masks

LED masks are usually futuristic plastic masks that contain LED panels or bulbs on the inside. You pop them onto your face for about ten minutes per day and let them do their work whilst you sit back and enjoy how Daft Punk you look. My favourite brand is Dermalux when it comes to professional LED therapy, but this is also a treatment that can be done at home.

In a study on the effectiveness of at-home LED masks undertaken in 2007 by Seun Yoon Lee at the National Medical Center in Seoul, it was found that, over a twelve-week period, inflammatory acne improved by 24.4 per cent when used daily. When you compare this to a study on LED

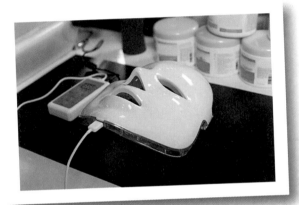

light therapy performed in a clinic in which there was a 77.9 per cent reduction by the end of an eight-week study, that is a whopping discrepancy in how effective it is.

On top of this, they must be used daily for ten minutes. Is a 24.4 per cent reduction in spots worth it for that much time? I guess that is up to the individual. What I can say is that an at-home mask can still have an effect and it is certainly a cost-effective method compared to professional LED therapy.

Professional Skincare Treatments

Professional treatments push the skin to work harder. Alongside a consistent homecare routine, they can help you to get results a little bit faster, especially if your skin concerns are more severe. If you're working to a deadline, like a graduation, your wedding day or just a goal you want to set for your own skin, a professional treatment can support your homecare in helping you to get where you want to be. These are a deeper workout and penetration of active ingredients.

Do you need salon treatments? Hell to the yes. But can you overdo it with salon treatments? Absolutely, especially with peels, and this is why a thorough consultation with a skincare professional that you trust is essential.

My personal go tos for professional treatments are:

HydraFacial MD (brand)

The HydraFacial is effectively a multi-step advanced treatment that is essentially suitable for all skin. It is a multi-modality treatment, meaning it is a cocktail of different treatments in one. It entails an exfoliation step that uses an AHA serum that is vacuum-blasted into the skin, a peel step with glycolic acid and salicylic acid, vacuum suction for extraction and an infusion step where serums are infused into the skin. It's a VIP, red-carpet treatment, and is more of a quick fix than a repairing treatment, in my opinion.

It's great because it dissolves sebaceous filaments, the little grey or white tips primarily found around the nose that are often confused with blackheads. It's also fabulous when you need an injection of moisture, such as when your skin just feels a bit 'meh' and your makeup isn't sitting well.

The exfoliation bit at the beginning is key as it sloughs off dead skin cells so that the following peel step can penetrate into the skin deeply and without any obstacles. The vacuum suction, as well as extracting debris from the pores, drains the lymphatic system to the relevant lymph nodes and increases blood circulation. It also releases oxygen onto the skin with a view to plumping the tissue and aiding in cell regeneration.

The HydraFacial needs literally no downtime and your skin will feel ridiculously soft to the touch, have high hydration levels and any blackheads will be gone.

I'd recommend this to people with sluggish, lethargic skin or someone looking to start a new skincare routine with a bang. It is not for sensitive or sensitised skin as it can be a bit abrasive, nor is it for those with active acne because of the possible spread of bacteria.

Microneedling

This is a treatment that uses fine needles, ranging in diameter from 1mm to 1.5mm, to reach the dermis and cause microtrauma and micro tears which trigger a cascade of collagen production. This is something that neither skincare, nor massaging, nor nutrition will be able to do and so this is an ideal treatment for anyone who suffers with a condition relating to collagen or elastin, such as lax pores, slackened jowls, loose skin around the eye region, forehead lines, redness and broken capillaries.

It is advisable to have it in a course because, as with all traumas to the skin, we can only do so much in one sitting. Usually you would go for three to six treatments, with a month or a month and a half between treatments. However, recent studies by various companies suggest that having treatments within a fourteen day period is superior to spreading them further out as it allows growth factors to peak and then continuously build up over time.

It is a treatment that has stood the test of time, but I do not trust all therapists to do well – and if it isn't done well, no collagen is triggered. Sometimes, therapists are heavy handed and trigger blood. Be aware of who you allow touch your face. Speak to friends who have had it done and talk about their result and where they went. Speak to your chosen therapist about their qualifications and the results that their clients have had with it. ITEC (globally recognised qualification) have a microneedling course and they are well-respected – however, usually therapists will learn to microneedle with the brand that their salon or clinic works with, for example, Dermapen or Nanopore. It comes down to technique, which is why hearing about others' results, reading reviews and asking the salon if you can see previous results they've had it so important.

Mesotherapy

Mesotherapy is the same concept as above and is often wrongly marketed as microneedling. The difference is that it's done using a 0.5mm needle so doesn't always reach the dermis and is more of a penetrant enhancer for large molecules such as hyaluronic acid. Mesotherapy, or meso needling, creates channels in the surface of the skin to allow products to get in.

Mesotherapy suits mature skin seeing as it is usually done with hyaluronic acid which plumps up and makes the skin look younger. The treatment is ideal for dull, sluggish skin in need of a bit of pepping up and dry or dehydrated skin in need of a moisture infusion.

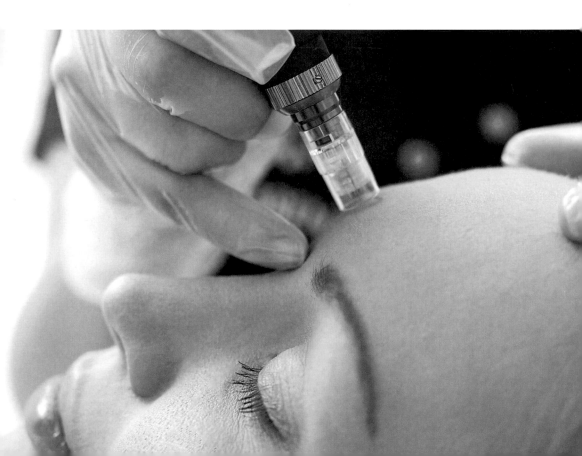

LED

LED (light emitting diode) was first developed by NASA when they were looking into how light would influence the growth of plants. Doctors decided it might be worth it to see if it would encourage dermal growth in skin.

LED treatments are a form of low-level light therapy (LLLT). The interesting thing about the skin being an organ is that it encounters light so much more frequently than any other organ in the body *yet* it still responds incredibly well to specific wavelengths of light. The skin can absorb light and convert it into energy. This energy stimulates a higher rate of cell turnover and aids in lymphatic drainage. A higher cell turnover rate equals fresher looking skin and better general skin health; an improved lymphatic drainage equals less puffiness and more radiancy – no more under-eye pillows, no more bloaty face, no more dullness or greyness.

Although LED phototherapy targets the dermal layer of the skin, every layer of the skin will benefit, so it is ideal for someone looking for a thorough skin rejuvenation.

There are three types of LEDs used in light-therapy facials and treatments: blue, red and near infrared. They work well separately but are also great together depending on your skin.

Blue light

Blue LED has been proven to successfully kill P. Acnes, the acne-causing bacteria that lives on the skin. It also calms irritation and inflammation.

Using blue light in acne treatment is effective because it is not 'hands on' per se, and so can successfully treat skin that is reactive and has possibly been subjected to trauma for years by using treatments like harsh exfoliation, microdermabrasion and strong peels.

Red light

When red light is emitted onto the skin, it can stimulate the fibroblast cell, which is the type of cell that makes up the connective tissue in the skin and synthesises collagen. This means it could be a game changer for those looking to improve the tone and texture of their skin in terms of anti-ageing. The reason that it is paired with the blue light in acne treatment is because it goes that bit deeper into the skin than the blue light and can also kill bacteria. They are a superhero duo, with the blue light battling the baddies further up in the skin and the red light getting the ones hiding in the shadows. The red light also brings down inflammation and swelling, shrinking them dastardly spots.

Near-infrared light

The near-infrared light can be absorbed most deeply into the skin and can aid in the skin's natural production of collagen, thus counteracting skin damage and the signs of ageing that the skin has already accumulated.

In the LED treatment, you're put under a little bridge of LED lights or a Daft Punk-style mask is popped on you usually for in and around twenty minutes.

Sometimes, LED phototherapy treatments are paired with peels and other treatments.

LED phototherapy is suitable for everybody and beneficial in some way or in another. There is no down time but, unlike the HydraFacial, you'd need to be having a full course of LED treatments to see a discernible difference, especially for acne and collagen synthesis (it can be from four to ten sessions). I would also advise having the treatments done in close proximity to each other, such as once a week. Having it once a month isn't quite worth it.

IPL

IPL, aka intense pulsed light, aka the photofacial is a treatment where multiple wavelengths of light are scattered across the skin. IPL is used to treat redness, broken capillaries, pigmentation from either sun damage or acne and in ageing skin to promote the production of collagen, as well as for hair removal.

It works like a spotlight on a stage to target a specific area and then emits wavelengths that target pigment (colouration of any kind). You may have heard before that IPL works best on those with lighter skin – this is because there needs to be a stark contrast between what the wavelengths are targeting and the skin itself for it to work. The IPL can't tell the difference between whether the colour is from the unaffected skin, from hair, from a spot of pigment or from a broken capillary so if the concern you're trying to target with IPL is too close in colour to your own skin tone, it may damage the skin itself.

The targeted light injures the tissue (or hair) that is causing the concern and the body gets rid of this injured tissue.

Regardless of why you're getting IPL, a cooling gel will be used and a cooling mechanism will be turned on on the machine. Otherwise, you'd feel like you were on fire as the wavelengths are going pretty deep in there to get to the follicle. IPL for hair removal isn't painful – it's like having a hot elastic band snapped against your skin.

However, IPL for redness diffusion and for blood vessels is supposedly a bit more painful but highly effective, so you win some, you lose some. In this case the cooling mechanism would make the whole treatment ineffective so it can't be used, hence the extra discomfort.

IPL for pigmentation can also use the cooling mechanism so it is more comfortable than IPL for redness diffusion and broken capillaries and the like.

If you're looking to use IPL for hair removal, it's usually recommended that you have six to twelve treatments. For pigmentation, depending on the severity, you could be looking at about four treatments and for redness diffusion and treatment of blood vessels and veins, it's usually around five treatments.

It's a treatment that has no downtime but you may see a bit of swelling, redness and soreness for a few hours up to a day after you've had it done.

Electrical muscle stimulation

Electrical muscle stimulation (EMS) is a passive form of exercise for the face where your muscles are stimulated using a wand that transfers microcurrents into your face. The microcurrents cause your muscles to intermittently contract and relax which tones the muscles in the same way that Slendertone machines do for other parts of your body. It's also known as CACI or Faradic.

Given that no topical skincare can even directly reach the dermis, no topical skincare can come anywhere near the muscles, which is why I think EMS is ace. Toned muscles prop up the skin, making it look plump and younger. There are no side-effects to EMS and your skin will look firmer immediately

It's for mature skin, but is preventative for anyone from the age of twenty-five. You can't use it if you have any issue with electricity going through your body, due to pregnancy, epilepsy, a pacemaker, etc. Always ask for or read instructions.

Ultherapy

Ultherapy is a clinical but non-invasive procedure where a wand that emits targeted ultrasound into the skin brings up the temperature of the tissues beneath the skin and heats them at different depths. This heating of the tissues means that the proteins within the skin change shape, triggering the healing cascade where masses of collagen are created to help to fix the 'wound' that the skin thinks has occurred.

It targets the SMAS (facial superficial musculoaponeurotic system), the structure that links your dermis and your epidermis, and so triggers the creation of collagen and elastin to make the skin tauter and plumper.

Ultherapy can lift the skin back up, as it works on its foundations rather than on its roof, per se. It's great for the dreaded 'turkey neck' and sagging jowls. As it is targeted, it passes through the other layers of the skin without causing harm and it can get deeper than any other technology. It requires no downtime. It depends on where you're getting it done but the face and neck procedure usually takes between sixty to ninety minutes. This is predominantly useful for anti-ageing, specifically structurally!

Iontophoresis

Iontophoresis is a treatment that involves electric current (galvanic charge) being pulsed into the skin for the purpose of helping products to penetrate deeper. This happens due to the movement of positive and negative ions (electrical charges) in the product itself. Iontophoresis is applied using a bar or wand or a flat stainless steel head that rotates across your face. In terms of sensation, it's not painful but there is a tingling, pins and needles feeling. If you have fillings, you can taste the metal in your mouth.

Not all products can be given a charge – they have to be able to conduct electricity. If you remember from science in school, oil cannot conduct electricity so oil-based products and ingredients are a no-go for iontophoresis.

Manufacturers provide a wide range of serums and gels to allow the iontophoresis machine and the serum to interact and attract together. This works on the premise of opposites attract. If the machine is set up on a negative pole, the serum will be that of a negative also as they will wish to be further away from one another. This means the serum that has been applied directly to the skin will have no choice but to be pushed into the lower layers of the skin.

This treatment is good for circulation and vasodilation (the dilating of blood vessels, which will help to diffuse redness in the skin) and generally ideal for improving the clarity of the skin.

Iontophoresis is for everybody, except those who can't have electrical current. You will have a pre-treatment consultation after which you will know whether or not you are suitable to have an electrical current treatment.

Direct high frequency

This treatment involves the use of a glass electrode which is moved slowly over the skin, warming the tissue underneath. The machine uses a high-frequency current, alternating with (very nerdie!) high-voltage low current. Unlike EMS, it won't contract the muscles as the pulses are too short. There are two kinds, direct and indirect. Direct high frequency is when the current is applied directly to the client's skin, whereas in indirect high frequency, the patient holds the electrode and the frequency gets into the whole body when the practitioner touches the skin of the client. Sound bananas? It kind of is but it's effective! Indirect high frequency improves circulation meaning more nutrients and oxygen to the individual skin cells. The resulting increased metabolic rate promotes the healing ability of the skin and the skin's vasodilation which increases blood flow and thus nutrients to the cells.

It feels just like a buzzing sensation with a bit of heat and, once again, if you have braces or fillings you may taste metal.

Direct is ideal for oilier and acne-prone skin as it has a germicidal, antibacterial, astringent (drying) effect.

Chemical peel

This is also known as an acid peel. All acids peels cause the skin to exfoliate at a much, much faster rate, which is what causes the redness after the treatment.

Peels consist of a high-percentage acid solution applied to the skin which is left for a period of time (usually just a few minutes, depending on the acid being used). Your skin will be thoroughly cleansed and prepped prior to your peel and you'll be sent home with a lovely layer of SPF on you to protect your slightly more susceptible skin.

The acids used in these peels are safe and will not destroy your skin as long as they are being administered by someone who has had training – using professional-grade peels at home is a very different story and something you should never do.

Your peel may be glycolic, lactic or salicylic based. Glycolic peels are best for those with dullness, sluggish-looking skin or those looking to get rid of hyperpigmentation. Lactic acid is best for those looking for something a bit more hydrating and gentle than a glycolic peel. Salicylic acid peels are best for the spot-prone.

You'll also find blends of different acids with enzymes and vitamins for multiple benefits at once. Your consultant or clinician will be able to advise you on what type of chemical peel will be best for you.

Chemical peels are ideal for those looking to deal with pigmentation, tonal issues, acne, ageing and scarring.

After a peel, your skin may be red and slightly irritated and swollen. You can't wear makeup for the following eight hours. You must also be extra vigilant with your sunscreen, although you should already be wearing it daily.

Depending on your skin, you may need between four and six peels for the best results.

What About Spa Facials?

Spa facials have their place. Due to the emphasis on modes of massage and aromatherapeutic products, it is a relaxing experience and can invigorate and re-energise dull, tired and stressed skin. Relaxation of the body and mind IS important for the skin. We've already discussed the effects of stress on the skin so I'd never write off anything that can help to reduce stress. However, the fluffier and puffier spa treatments can't bring change to the lower levels of the skin. They can boost your skin's circulation, help with lymphatic drainage and maybe exfoliate a bit if they're using acids but little else can be done from them.

Get spa facials if you want them – I love them too but they serve a different purpose to many of the other treatments I get. Just remember that results-driven salon and clinical facials are often more effective when it comes to skin health.

They're not all 'fluff puff' now either. Spa brands are bringing in modalities to manipulate tissue and stimulate circulation so they're bringing blood and oxygen to the area, toning the muscle and having anti-ageing effects. They have upped their game and they definitely have a place within the skincare industry – it just depends on personal preferences

Finding a Therapist

People shouldn't be doing peels without ITEC, VTCT, CIBTAC or CIDESCO certifications in beauty therapy or advanced skincare so ask about that in the salon. Look up reviews and feel out for word of mouth recommendations among your skin-savvy friends. If you come across a salon that you haven't heard a lot about but want to give a try anyway, ensure that they carry out a detailed consultation, asking about your skin's past and present, and your future goals. Questions should be plentiful, thorough and explained. A plan of action should be decided, including a mutually agreed realistic timeline.

A good consultation means that you'll be encouraged to explain everything about your skin rather than just required to put down your name and signature and jump into a practised retail spiel. Rather than you simply saying 'my skin is oily' and being given a salicylic cleanser, in a thorough consultation, you'll be asked where the oiliness appears, if anything has changed in your life or skin of late, if you are exfoliating and other questions in this vein. Maybe the answer will be that you were actually over-exfoliating so you might be advised to stop exfoliating for a while, after which the consultant will put you on a new skincare routine. The difference is that you and your skin are prioritised over making a sale there and then. Rapport is essential and once you trust your advisor, keep them!

You are the client, you deserve to be knowledgeable after the time with your skin specialist.

Full Body Skin

In case I've given you the wrong impression, skin doesn't just appear on our face. It's a full body situation and as such, we need to consider not just facial skincare but everywhere else too. Here I will give an overview on skin beyond the face, common issues and things to be mindful of.

Neck and Décolletage

First up, do we treat our neck and chest the same way we treat our face?

Yes, we should. One of our catchphrases at Nerd HQ is 'nipples up'. This is something I heard years ago and it has stayed with me ever since. What we mean by saying this is that the tissue on the neck, décolletage and upper breasts can defy time and gravity if attention is given to them. So, make sure that you don't forget about these areas when it comes to skincare. Your face, neck and decolletage are a delicate area of thinner skin than the rest of your body and they are the most likely to be exposed to sun on a regular basis so they deserve slightly better treatment.

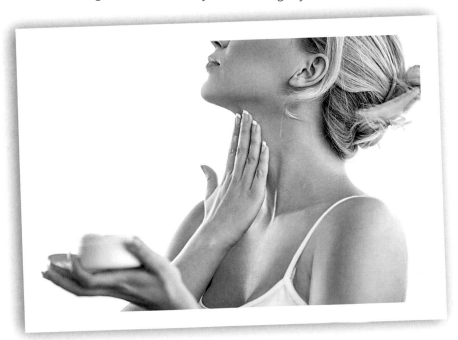

Hands

The hands give our age away as we usually never apply sunscreen, antioxidants or any other products to them so my advice would be to pump out a little more product than is necessary for the face, neck and décolletage, applying the excess to the back of the hands. Definitely make a point of applying SPF to the hands.

If you want to go one step further, use an acid-infused hand cream for super soft hands like Murad Rejuvenating AHA Hand Cream. For hands that are showing signs of ageing, opt for IPL or apply a lightening treatment such as the Neostrata Enlighten Pigment Lightening Gel. And wear gloves when doing mundane household chores.

Lips

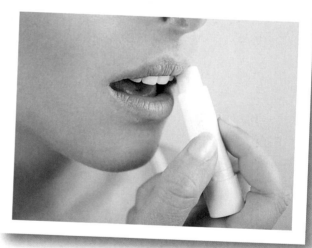

Lips need care too – it is also skin. We should be using SPF lip balm on the daily and exfoliating them mildly with a mix of coconut oil and a fine sugar. Those with cold sores should take care when it comes to lip scrubs as physical trauma to your lips can trigger a cold sore. Supplement L-Lysine is particularly good for cold sores, but if they are a regular occurrence for you, consult your doctor.

Most serums can be applied to your lips, so don't go out of your way to avoid the lips when applying. Avoid acid usage on lips if you get cold sores, some have found that it can trigger them – the heat or inflammation caused can set up the virus. We eat our lips and lick them so be mindful of them as they are made up of a reactive response membrane.

Everywhere Else

Supplements (p.79) and body brushing are two modes of looking after the skin across your whole body. Acid-based exfoliators are just as important for the body as for the 'nipples up' area, especially for those with spots on their body and keratosis pilaris (see below).

You should exfoliate your whole body – bar any areas that you wouldn't want to put an acid exfoliant on, if you get what I mean. No scrubs though. Mechanical exfoliation causes micro-tears to the skin, especially cumulatively, so opt for acid-based or enzyme-based body lotions and exfoliators.

You can exfoliate your body once or twice a week and that should be enough. I'd also recommend doing it after you shave or wax to prevent ingrown hairs, as it will clear the dead skin cells from blocking the now shorter hair's way.

What's Keratosis Pilaris?

Those little blocked, spot-like buggers you'll find on the backs of your arms and legs. KP is usually found on the back of the arms but it can manifest itself on any part of the body. In appearance, it looks a bit like pixelated skin; very small reddish, pinkish or flesh-coloured dots that cover the affected area.

You're most likely to find it on women and, surprisingly, children! If keratin is overproduced within the pore, it can become trapped there, rather than moving outwards with the shedding dead skin cells as it usually does. This causes a 'traffic jam' within the pore, leading to keratosis pilaris.

Unfortunately, this tendency to overproduce keratin is passed on from generation to generation, meaning that if you have keratosis pilaris, you have it for good.

Taking Vitamin A and omegas orally could be the step you need to add to your life to banish the bumps! It is believed that Vitamin A may have a hand in correcting the keratinisation process, stopping the follicles from becoming plugged in the first place, by actually slowing down the rate in which the skin gets rid of dead skin cells due to the skin cells being able to function longer.

Glycolic acid is keratolytic meaning it softens keratin and helps the body to shed dead skin cells. For this reason lotions and treatments that contain glycolic acid can help, as can salicylic acid which dissolves the plug of dead skin cells and exfoliates the skin. Lactic acid is also highly effective.

Hydration and skin health is also key for keratosis pilaris so many find sanctuary from KP in vitamin-enriched lotions and ones that contain hyaluronic acid.

KP is one of the most common conditions out there, and probably the reason that Irish women love cardigans so much; it's very normal and nothing to be overly concerned about.

What about particularly dry/scaly legs? Very dry, scaly skin on legs is a sign of a deficiency of essential fatty acids. Boost them through taking supplements and eating more fish, nuts, seeds and oils. If it's an ongoing issue and happens in patches, take yourself to the GP as it could be a more serious skin issue, especially if it's itchy and causing you pain.

Cellulite

Cellulite is, perhaps, the biggest concern most people have when it comes to full body skin concerns. It occurs is when fatty packets protrude into the skin's tissues, causing the dimpled, puckered effect that you see on the skin's surface. It is not something that can be eradicated or prevented per se – we all have fat on our bodies – literally all of us – and this is what fat may do.

It is not something that happens because you are carrying extra weight either.

Contrary to popular belief, cellulite is more than normal. It is especially common in women because of their physiological makeup. Women's connective tissue, just above their subcutaneous fat, has larger openings in it which makes it easier for these fatty protrusions to get through. It is especially common on bums, tums and thighs – which are the areas that are naturally fattier on women. Genetics definitely play a role with regard to cellulite too.

Grades of cellulite

Grade 1: Cellulite is never visible, even when the skin is manipulated.

Grade 2: Cellulite is visible when the skin is pinched or pressed together, but the skin appears cellulite-free when you're standing upright.

Grade 3: The cellulite can be seen whilst standing but is not visible when you are lying down flat.

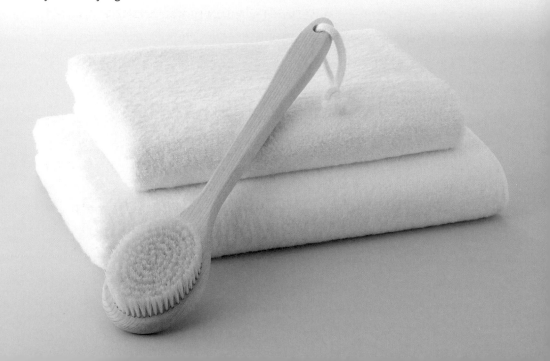

Grade 4: Dimpling and puckering is always easily visible but appears worse when the skin is pinched.

What clients hate to hear is that you can never fully get rid of cellulite, but the good news is there are things you can do to improve its appearance, including body brushing and massage.

Body brushing improves circulation, helps lymphatic drainage and keeps your skin hydrated. It won't get rid of cellulite, or really affect it at all, but hydrated skin shows fewer flaws so it will definitely be less noticeable if you're moisturising.

Any cream that claims to actually fix cellulite is lying. A cream cannot get to the dermis, so ignore its siren call.

Many also see an effect from manual massage of the areas. Endermologie Lipomassage, which uses suction to stimulate lymphatic drainage and circulation and aids in the body's own production of collagen, is a good one to try.

VelaShape, which targets the fat cells directly using thermal energy (infrared light and bipolar radio frequency), also uses mechanical massage and suction. Like Lipomassage, it also helps with lymphatic drainage, circulation and boosts collagen production. VelaShape also uses radiofrequency for tissue tightening and increased circulation, both of which will help to reduce the appearance of cellulite.

What else can you do?

None of us want to hear this but keeping toned helps to reduce the appearance of cellulite. Aim to work out two to three times per week and have a twenty-minute walk per day. This gets the lymphatic system going and improves circulation.

Avoid processed foods. Eating healthy food rich in antioxidants, vitamins and minerals doesn't help with cellulite directly. However, eating nutrient-rich foods helps our bodies to create collagen to its best advantage and aids skin cells in protecting themselves. Your connective tissue needs protein to feed it so get enough protein in your diet to back it up.

In general, you need to see food as fuel and remember that what you put in is what you get out. Whole foods are always going to be better for you. Where possible, your food should be things you can find in nature. I haven't seen cake hanging from a tree lately – although I wish I had – have you?

To sum up, body brushing is the most effective way to lightly exfoliate and trigger the sluggish lymphatic system. Always move the soft bristles towards the heart and do it daily before you shower.

Out of the Ordinary

Skincare for Special Occasions

As The Skin Nerd, I'm all about optimal skincare all day every day but, for special occasions – brides and grooms-to-be in particular – there are a few extra things you can do. I've used the example of preparing for a wedding in the following guide, but these steps will be applicable to any big event that you're working towards.

When to start

When planning your outfit, psyche yourself up for the skin regime at the same time. Many wait until six weeks before their big day to think about their skin and this may not be enough time to tackle any true concerns. I always say to people, as soon as your engagement party is over, book your consult.

If you're looking to clear up stubborn things that take time like pigmentation prior, you need to have time on your side and, by time, I mean at least six months to a year (preferably).

The average skin cycle is a month and you need to be using some products for a few cycles to see a real change, specifically things like Vitamin A and lightening products.

What not to do

Don't throw the kitchen sink at your skin just because you are getting married – there is such thing as too much. Using more acids will speed up your cell turnover. But using too many can impair your barrier leading to scaliness, redness and even painful breakouts. You need to be under guidance at all times.

If you're considering microneedling (see page 247), which helps for dull, lethargic skin, sagging skin, fine lines, scars and pigmentation, you should aim to do it six months before the big day and no sooner. For peels

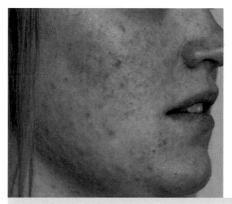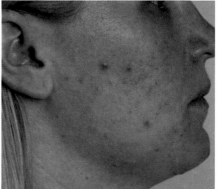

Some people don't see that their skin needed TLC. This client wanted her skin to be smoother and plumper with less inflammation. As you can see, her skin looks healthier in the second photo, just in time for her wedding.

or IPL, three months before the day should be OK. Don't try anything you've not tried before within a month of your wedding unless advised to do so by your facialist.

In that final month, don't introduce new products or ingredients into your homecare routine either – to be on the super-safe side, keep your routine nearly exactly the same in the last two months leading up to your day. I tend to up the ante for brides' skin but I'll only introduce ingredients that they have tried previously.

You don't want to have any adverse reactions or cause harm to your skin's barrier in the lead up to your big day in case it proves difficult to counteract in such a short space of time. It will also cause undue stress which you certainly won't need.

Planning a wedding is a stressful process so you need to wrap yourself in cotton wool a bit and make sure you're all right.

What should change?

Planning a wedding can be an extremely busy time so be sure to up the multivitamin intake. Horse the Vitamin C into you – 1000mg daily – to warn off colds while also strengthening your capillary walls. Bear in mind that red is the first colour to be seen on camera! I'd also recommend taking lysine, an amino acid that assists the virus that is herpes simplex to prevent cold sores.

Take omegas internally (i.e. essential fatty acids) in the form of supplements or oily fish. These will have your body wedding and honeymoon ready – helping keep it soft with less inflammation and fewer stress breakouts. If you don't already have a skincare regime that works for you, it is at that six-month to go mark that you should get on one as recommended through a thorough consult.

Then, do everything else listed for healthy skin throughout this book.

Sample Bride/Groom-to-Be Special Event Skincare Schedule	
12 months	• Have a consultation, if you haven't already. • Start taking supplements – Vitamin A, omega and Vitamin C, as well as using a consistent home routine full of active products. • If you're looking to have a course of treatments done to clear up any concerns, you can do one now and then protect the skin vigilantly with SPF and tyrosinase-inhibiting products until your big day.
9 months	• Have a follow-up consultation about your home routine, if you haven't already. • If you think you'd like to change something in your routine or maybe up the ante a smidge, this is the time to discuss it.
6 months	• If you're hoping to do a bit of microneedling, start it now.

3 months	• Peels should be done now, same for IPL. I'm a big fan of the Neostrata Rejuvenating Peel. Consider your décolletage, upper arms, back and anywhere else your garment may be exposing. • Keep your home care the same from now on. • If you are having a wax for the event, go for a patch test now. Waxperts wax leaves no redness and will give you fuzz-free limbs for the big day!
1 month	• As a rule of thumb, don't change your home-care routine, unless you are being guided. Hyaluronic acid is A-OK to add in. • Reduce your sugar intake. • Do not have any treatments unless you know your therapist well and they know your skin. • Do not pop any spots (to prevent post-inflammatory hyperpigmentation). • Start looking after your body skin if you haven't already – start exfoliating your body skin with acid-based exfoliators and body brushing.
1 week	• Avoid laser treatments. • Get your Waxperts wax done at least a full week before the wedding (if you are getting a wax). • Get your spray tan done two days prior to the big day and make sure to exfoliate thoroughly with an acid-based body lotion, like IMAGE Skincare Body Spa Rejuvenating Lotion. • Make sure you're using hyaluronic acid regularly to keep your skin plump and fresh. • Prep the hands – if you're getting married, they'll be shown off in photos of your bouquet, the signing of the register and the ring exchange.

Night before	• Skip your usual spot treatments to avoid cornflaking of spots. • Slather any scabbing or spots in your usual soothing, hydrating product. • Do an overnight masque if there is already one in your routine. • Drink plenty of water! • Sleep!
Day of	• Use a mild cleanser. • Apply calming serums. • Hold cold spoons under your eyes for instant constriction of blood vessels to reduce under-eye puffiness – this actually works, but only temporarily • If you have an EMS machine or the Environ Electro Sonic DF Mobile Device, use this in the morning while bridesmaids are being looked after. • Prior to applying your makeup, pop on a tackier, stickier serum or SPF to give your makeup something to adhere to. • Enjoy your beautiful skin and your big day!

Taking Your Skin on Holiday

Unfortunately your skin doesn't really take holidays – sorry! – but here are a couple of tips that will help you mind your skin when you're away from home.

- When travelling, it's very important to take care of your skin – and you can achieve this in a few different ways.

  - Before you leave for your trip, don't forget to consume essential fatty acids/fish oils to keep the skin's moisture levels up. This means the skin is plumped and protected against the elements, and can resist the negative effects of in-flight air conditioning.

- Use a water spritz to keep your skin hydrated throughout your journey.
- Decant your favourite hydrating mask into a travel-sized pot to treat your skin and use cooling anti-inflammatory eye pads to keep this delicate, think-skinned area hydrated – go on, be that diva!
- Drinking water won't do much for the skin by itself, but it is vital to hydrate cells.
- If you wear makeup, keep it minimal.
- Wear breathable, cotton clothing so the skin is not chafed and irritated while seated for long periods.
- Wear SPF – UVA rays beam through the windows of cars, trains and planes!
- When you arrive, use a gentle exfoliating product to lift the debris, dry skin and excess oil from the surface of the skin.

- When on holiday, be safe when it comes to the sunshine! Cover up as much as possible and regardless of your SPF's factor or your skin colour, reapply every two hours. (And in case you thought you didn't need SPF on winter holidays, you're wrong!)

- If you're spending a lot of time in the water, keep your skin moisturised – and remember to keep topping up on that sunscreen!

- Antioxidants fight against the free radicals from the sun, food and drinks we may be exposed to while in holiday mode, so applying them topically under your SPF every day is essential.

- Exfoliation is key (but remember not to do this excessively!)

- You might be tempted to ignore your skincare regime but please don't

– your skin needs to be minded more than ever! What you could do is scale back slightly to your daily cleanser, your serum and SPF as well as any treatments you use regularly.

Skin Diary Check-in:

- *Have you been filling out your skin diary? Have you done your homework ? Uh-oh! Now that you're clued in in all things nerdie about the skin, it's time to do an overall mini-analysis on yourself, using all the details you've noted so far and all the information you've learned. Crack out your magnifying glass, Nancy Drew.*

- *What's your sleep looking like? How many times do you get less than seven hours sleep? Is it 10 per cent of the time? Is it once per week? Is it more than 50 per cent of the time? If it's more than 50 per cent of the time, that could be your culprit for dullness and dark circles.*

- *Check the days that you marked that you ate lots of sugar and measure them against what your skin was like in the following day. Were there more breakouts? Interestingly it can be twenty-eight days later that you see some agents of lifestyle change as this is the skin we see that is a result of the health at the lower layers one month prior. So prolonged stress can become visible one month post illness / post medication etc. if only it was at the time; I know!*

- *When you marked your stress levels as higher or lower, check to see what your skin was like in the time around this. It could potentially be sluggish, grey, dull in appearance, somewhat lacklustre and in dire need of nutrition. As we now know the skin is an organ! It will be devoid of plentiful nutrition if the vital organs have required it. I personally find my skin's healing ability to be less i.e. blemishes remain and the texture is rougher to the touch. Each person aka hooman is different and the diary helps you to discover your own pattern.*

- *Some may think of stress and think of something dramatic such as a bereavement or major money issues when a simple example for me would be on the last Wednesday of each month when I have a large management meeting for the company in which I prepare all financials, vision, press summaries, etc. It is full on! I am always so prepared for it that I wouldn't describe it as a stressful meeting – yet our bodies know better than us sometimes. I monitored my skin for three months and learned my skin's behaviour around this monthly meeting. Similarly I travel long distances the first week of the month and monitor my skin's reaction to the heat in the car and again I began to see a rhythm. The good news is I tweaked my supplements and skincare to boost immunity and the result the following month was visible; this is the beauty of the diary. It puts you in the driving seat. You can't change the destination (as sometimes stress or other things affecting our skin are unavoidable) but you can help the body's means of coping with it.*

- *This is key for you to know your triggers, unique to you, especially if you're prone to breakouts or redness and to create changes to your skincare approach – whether that's exploring treatment options, adding an additional step to your nightly routine, or making sure that you've always got a mini bottle of SPF in your handbag – that suit your skin and your life.*

And keep filling in your diary – it's a valuable tool in your skincare journey, and will help you track what's helping and what might need changing. Keep it by your bed (along with your copy of this book!) and update it regularly to help it help you.

Conclusion

Thank you for reading – you are officially an honorary Nerd. You now have the basis of a wealth of skinformation. You understand why peptides, antioxidants and Vitamins A and C are key, why you have to pre-cleanse before you cleanse and why it is blasphemous to purposefully not wear SPF. You know the touch and feel of your skin; you know it inside out.

You now – I hope! – look at your skin as an organ. You respect it (think of this every time you shower!). You're committed to investing in effective skingredients that will assist it to be as healthy as it can be. It can be a barometer for internal health. It certainly provides you with an opportunity to take five minutes both night and day to mind you. You are important.

You are now ready to take your first steps on the path to optimal skin health – go you!

Be savvy, smell less and lean on the education! Become a nerd and identity the aspects you'd like to change – it's OK to not want pigmentation or broken capillaries. It's not vanity; it's the opposite – it's identifying how we can feed the skin with more goodness than what it currently receives and allow it to be the healthy ambassador for you as it should be.

Remember, a thorough consultation is always advisable – as are follow-up consultations – as we are emotionally attached to ourselves and so it can be tough to objectively see what's really going on with our skin.

Skin always changing, no routine should be set in stone for a long period of time, and because of this, regular consultations are smart. Your skin is a dynamic, living (but not breathing) thing. It changes like everything else in life – it changes when you age, when the seasons change, when your lifestyle changes, if you get pregnant, if you are going through the menopause.

What's more, every single person's skin is different, or skindividual, as we like to say here at Nerd HQ. Ingredients that I've recommended for a condition may not suit your skin for certain reasons unbeknownst to me. You need an outsider to look at your skin, specifically a qualified outsider, someone who will look at your skin objectively.

Education is key and there is a lot of miseducation and biased education out there. Someone at a one-brand stall in a shopping centre is going to sell you that brand and that brand only. So please be mindful of this. That's not to say this isn't the right recommendation for you, but use your Nerdie book-smart wisdom to challenge their suggestions.

To Do Straight After Reading

- Throw out wipes and micellar water #binthewipes.

- Cut down on caffeine intake (AHEM including tea, not just coffee) – get the water in to you.

- Ditch the scrubs – even the body ones; seek out the acids. Because the skin is acidic, it accepts them better.

- Each day, breathe in and out deeply for sixty seconds as you are cleansing your face. See this as 'me time'.

- Every day, pre-cleanse, cleanse, use serum and SPF.

- Try and avoid the marketing hype, please and thank you.

- Investigate the back of the bottles and see what ingredients you have already in your cabinet

- Book a consultation!

- See skincare as a jigsaw puzzle; be patient with it.

- Enjoy your skin – see it, treat it and respect it as an organ.

- Be you, always.

Jennifer

 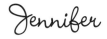

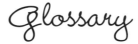

Glossary

Acid mantle – aka the skin's barrier. A thin, acidic coating on the surface of our skin that protects from bacteria and debris and keeps moisture in.

Amino acids – compounds that make up protein, which can be found in food, our skin and skingredients (such as peptides).

Androgens – a male sex hormone, e.g. testosterone.

Antioxidants – compounds that stop oxidation from occurring. In the context of skin, they protect it by neutralising free radicals.

Bioavailability – the rate and amount of which something can be successfully absorbed by the body.

Cell membrane – the semipermeable protective layer around the cell (which lets good substances in and keeps bad ones out).

Circadian rhythm – the sleep/wake cycle, which keeps us awake when we need to be awake and asleep when we should be asleep.

Collagen – the most abundant protein found in the body, gives skin its strength and structure along with elastin.

Comedones – skin-coloured small bumps usually found on the head or chin if acne is an issue. Blackheads are known as open comedones as they do not have a covering of skin, whiteheads are known as closed comedones as they <u>do</u> have a covering of skin!

Comedogenic – if a substance or ingredient clogs pores, it is comedogenic or a comedogen.

Cortisol – a slow-releasing stress hormone that is a part of many different functions within the body.

Cosmeceutical – a combination of the words 'cosmetic' and 'pharmaceutical', relating to skincare products. Cosmeceutical products are predominantly filled with highly active ingredients such as alpha-hydroxy acids, Vitamin A and others. The majority of cosmeceutical products are accessed through consultation only, although this is slowly changing.

Desquamation – scientific term for skin's natural exfoliation process, when the dead skin cells on the very top of the epidermis shed off.

Digestive Enzymes – specific enzymes that make digestion a lot easier on your gut, such as lactase, lipase and bromelain.

Eczema – a skin condition thought to have genetic factors as well as extrinsic (environmental) factors. Eczema appears as itchy, flaky, scaly, red and inflamed skin and it differs in severity. Many believe that the immune system is overzealous about tackling what it perceives to be a threat and thus the physical symptoms occur.

EFAs – Essential Fatty Acids, required for regulation of skin cell membranes, incredibly helpful at reducing inflammation and necessary for the skin's barrier function.

Elastin – protein that is responsible for skin's elasticity; ensures that our skin snaps to our bodily contours so that we are not just a bag of bones.

Electron – a subatomic particle that carries a negative electric charge.

Enzyme – a substance produced by a living organism that acts as a catalyst to bring about a specific biochemical reaction in the body. Essentially, they help to speed up chemical reactions throughout the body. When it comes to skincare, enzymes are used topically as a mild, sensitive-skin-friendly exfoliant to gobble off dead skin cells like Pac Man.

Free radical – an atom or molecule with an unpaired electron that frantically tries to find something to attach itself to, causing damage to cellular structures in the process. In the skin, they cause accelerated ageing.

Glycemic index – a scale that measures how quickly blood sugar levels rise after eating a particular food.

Gut-skin axis – how gut health influences skin health.

Homeostasis – consistent balance, within a body's systems.

Humectant – something that holds onto moisture well and draws moisture to it, either up from the lower layers of the skin or in from the air.

Hyperpigmentation – when melanin is overproduced in a particular area of the skin. Examples include age spots/sun spots and acne marks (post-inflammatory hyperpigmentation).

Hypopigmentation – a loss of pigment (melanin) in the skin; it often appears as white patches.

Insulin – an important hormone that regulates your blood sugar levels.

Keratin – the protein that is a key constituent of our skin, hair and nails.

Keratinisation – the process in which skin cells become horny (as in filled with keratin, not what you're thinking) and move upwards through the epidermis.

Keratinocyte Cell – the 'mother cell' when found in the basal layer of the skin as they divide to create other cells, they make up 90% of the epidermis.

Keratosis pilaris – aka 'chicken skin' – small flesh-coloured or pink bumps that look like pixelated skin, they occur due to an overproduction of keratin and a subsequent trapping of it in the pore.

Lax pores – pores that have lost their elasticity and widened.

Lentigos – a pigment mark or patch of pigment that develops due to exposure to UV rays, e.g. age spots, liver spots (also known as lentigines).

Lipids – fats, essential component of living cells. Lipids are insoluble in water (hydrophobic).

Lymphatic system – the system of lymph vessels that transports lymph (a clear fluid) towards your heart and helps us to get rid of toxins.

Melanin – a pigmen that gives our skin cells, eyes and hair colour. This is what makes some of us naturally darker-skinned than others, and what over-accumulates where we see hyperpigmentation occur.

Melanocyte cells – these make pigment, found in the basal layer of the skin within the epidermis.

Melasma – a mask or large patch formation of pigmentation, usually across the nose, cheeks, over the upper lip or on the forehead. In pregnancy, it is referred to as chloasma specifically.

Milia – small, hardened, round, pearly bumps, visibly deeper than a whitehead, most commonly found around the eye area but can be found anywhere across the body. They occur when oil and dead skin cells become trapped in the outer layers of the skin.

Mitochondria – a cell's engine room, the 'powerhouse of the cell', creates cellular energy.

Mitosis – the process in which cells are made when a cell divides and creates 'daughter cells'.

Monosaccharide – simple sugars, such as glucose, that cannot be hydrolyzed to be made any simpler. They help to build disaccharides (lactose, sucrose) and polysaccharides (cellulose, starch, beta-glucan).

Non-comedogenic – the opposite to comedogenic. If a substance is non-comedogenic, it doesn't clog pores.

Nucleus – the 'brain of the cell', the part of the cell that holds the genes of a cell and so controls its growth and reproduction.

OTC – over the counter - e.g. skincare that you can obtain freely without the need for a consultation with an expert.

Oxidation – the name for the process of something becoming oxidised, or when a substance gains oxygen. Rusting is caused by oxidation as is the browning of an apple that is left exposed without its skin. In the skin, oxidation causes free radical damage.

Oxidative Stress – what happens within the skin when there are too many free radicals and not enough antioxidants to balance them. It is oxidative stress that causes damage to cellular structures within the skin, accelerating the degradation of our collagen and elastin.

P. acnes – propionibacterium acnes, a primarily helpful bacteria that naturally lives on the skin but can cause congestion to become inflamed when it gets into the pore.

Peptides – amino acids holding hands. In skincare, they often send prompts for the skin to create collagen (amongst other things). Each peptide does something different and not all peptides are necessarily beneficial to the skin.

Photodamage – any damage that occurs to the skin due to exposure to UVA and UVB rays.

Photosensitise – to make the skin more sensitive to the effects of UVA or UVB rays so that it can become damaged more easily.

Phytonutrient – compounds found in plants that are not essential to humans but can have beneficial effects regardless. Examples of phytonutrients are carotenoids, flavonoids, resveratrol, lycopene and lutein.

Polyphenols – plant compounds that hunt down free radicals.

Pores – the opening of hair follicles, the tiny 'holes' across the surface of our skin that allow sebum to reach the surface of the skin, as they contain our sebaceous glands, the glands that create sebum.

Probiotics – living organisms that allow bacteria to colonise (in our gut, when ingested, or on the surface of the skin when applied topically) and restore natural bacterial balance.

Progesterone – a sex hormone that plays a role in pregnancy and the menstrual cycle, shown to have an effect on skin density and collagen production, amongst other things, when it drops due to menopause.

Proliferation – your skin's natural exfoliation process, the process of new skin cells being formed and others being sloughed off.

Psoriasis – an autoimmune disease that is characterised by red, itchy plaques covered in silvery scales of skin. Skin cells are created too rapidly and so the skin has to frantically try to get rid of dead skin cells even though they are not quite ready to slough off. This means that those 'not quite ready' dead skin cells are left to accumulate on the surface of the skin, forming plaques.

Rosacea – an auto-inflammatory skin disease that is associated with redness and flushing of the skin. There are four subtypes of rosacea and the exact cause is unknown.

Sebaceous gland – the gland that produces sebum within each pore.

Sebum – the skin's oils, or the oily secretion that comes from the sebaceous glands, made up of lipids such as triglycerides and squalene. It is part of our skin's protective acid mantle, makes us waterproof and lubricates our skin.

Sensitisation – the process of the skin becoming more sensitive to ingredients and products due to extrinsic factors or factors within your control, such as over-exfoliation, super hot showers, neglecting to use sunscreen and skin dehydration.

Squalane – what we get when we hydrogenate squalene (an ingredient of our skin's own oils/sebum), making it stable and giving it a longer shelf-life.

Sudoriferous glands – sweat glands.

Synthesise – to create more of something, to produce something through combining different elements.

Transepidermal water loss – when the skin's moisture is lost through the epidermis, the skin's barrier protects us from this when it is functioning properly.

Triglycerides – a lipid found throughout the body, helps to make up our sebum alongside squalane and fatty acids.

Tyrosinase inhibitors – ingredients that stop the production of tyrosinase (an enzyme that tells the skin to create melanin).

UVA rays – the ultraviolet rays emitted from the sun that are longer than UVB rays and thus can damage the skin at a deeper level than UVB rays - they can get to us through clouds and windows all year round. UVA rays, like UVB rays, play a role in the development of skin cancer.

UVB rays – the ultraviolet rays emitted from the sun that are shorter than UVA rays, the rays that cause sunburn, closely associated with skin cancer. They are predominant in the summer months.

Wax esters – ester of a fatty acid and a fatty alcohol, type of lipid found in our skin's sebum.

Image permissions

Acknowledgements

To my rocks, my mammy and daddy. Mammy, my childhood library chauffeur – my hope is for a dusty, battered and loved version of this book to feature on a library floor in the future! Dreams do come true and you founded mine. Daddy, my original proof-reader and the most meticulous one at that! You always say to read all documents twice and I certainly hope the nerdie readers will heed that advice! You're my inspiration and the reason why nerdiness is what I aspired to. Always.

To Matthew, my Mini Nerd – let's hope this inspires you to remain book-smart.

Thanks to everyone on Team Hachette, it was an honour to have been asked to write this book and the direction given in each and every step of the way has been truly appreciated.

To Caroline Foran, editor and nerdie translator extraordinaire; your inquisitive brain has moulded this skin bible into a reality. You are a consummate professional and bestselling author. I truly could not have asked for better guidance.

To Lucy Bennett, my right-hand word nerd. A truly thorough, dedicated writer who researches scrupulously to guarantee content of the highest calibre. This would not have been a possibility without your constant support. Please know that.

To Clare Muir, my professional skinspiration and mentor. It is you who encouraged me to have skin wisdom beyond the industry norm. Your brain is enviable and your yearning to learn motivates me massively. Thank you for all that you do for our industry. You may not see it but we all benefit from it greatly.

To Amy Buckeridge of Publicity Loft, my agent, PR ninja, professional rock and close friend. Thank you for taking my phone calls at all hours and for all that you do on a daily basis.

To Team Nerd, thank you for always having my back and for assisting with the pictures and clients. Charlotte, Hailey, Shannon and Robyn, you rock!

To the clients who allowed us to use their pictures, it means so much to be able to reinforce our message. Thank you for your time and your belief in our philosophy.

To those of you who have read this book, thank you for reading and I hope it will be something you can return to whenever you have a skin query.

Jennifer